# The NFL Guide
## to
# Physical Fitness

# The NFL Guide to Physical Fitness

## BY THE COACHES, DOCTORS, AND TRAINERS OF THE NATIONAL FOOTBALL LEAGUE

Edited by Richard Pickens

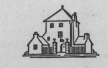

RANDOM HOUSE

Library of Congress Catalog Card Number: 65-11298

Manufactured in the United States of America

# THE NFL GUIDE TO PHYSICAL FITNESS

## FOREWORD

The amazing growth of the National Football League has provided an exciting spectacle for sports-loving Americans. As a former professional athlete, I know that we serve as a model of physical fitness for young and old alike.

It was with great interest that I read the *NFL Guide to Physical Fitness,* which has many helpful suggestions for Americans to keep themselves physically fit.

I appreciate the efforts of the National Football League for lending their support to this publication in the vital area of physical fitness for our citizens. I am sure this book will be well received.

*Stan Musial,*

Stan Musial
Consultant to the President
on Physical Fitness

October 1964

# CONTENTS

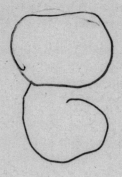

# THE BOOK'S PURPOSE

The National Football League player is the epitome of the American athlete — in size, speed, strength, and physical condition. The average player is 26.3 years old, stands 6 feet, 1.8 inches tall, and is 222.7 pounds of coordinated muscle and bone. Few men compare with this superb physical specimen, nor would the average young man be willing to undergo the hours of rigorous training required to enable him to perform in such a violent contact sport. Fortunately, few of us ever have to withstand the impact of a charging 250-pound lineman.

But *any* man can harden his muscles, sharpen his reflexes, and improve both his appearance and sense of physical well-being — by following consistently an intelligent program of exercise. This book offers you the same guiding principles as those used by NFL coaches and trainers in their conditioning of the best football players in the world. Equally important, it offers you a concept of physical fitness whose keynote is *flexibility*. For we believe that no matter how excellent a general exercise program may be, all men were created *unequal* — in that no two sets of muscles, pairs of arms or legs, or degrees of strength, speed, or resiliency are identical. Thus, a truly effective physical fitness program must not be general, but tailor-made to the needs of the individual. It must look beyond the necessary ingredient of exercise and consider the equally important factors of a man's age, occupation, body structure, and the level of physical capacity he may wish to attain — whether he be a rugged 200-pounder hoping to become a professional athlete, or a middle-aged businessman whose most violent activity is a fast game of ping-pong.

With an investment of time, patience, and energy, virtually any man can develop a better-looking body, greater

3

strength, endurance, and suppleness, and can wake up in the morning feeling confident and optimistic.

By putting emphasis on personal factors, *we have designed this book to help you "custom build" a program of physical fitness for yourself.* By following its principles and advice sensibly, you can attain that level of condition best suited to your body and to your personal goals.

## YOUR DOCTOR'S ROLE

We strongly urge that you get a complete physical examination before starting any physical fitness program. In addition to its precautionary value, a clean bill of health is of great psychological value. And we suggest that you discuss your entire planned program with your doctor, for he may be able to make suggestions that will help you considerably on your road to physical fitness.

*If you have any physical difficulties, injuries, or have suffered any kind of illness, it is absolutely imperative for you to work closely with your doctor.*

There is a great deal of difference between a physical fitness program for a healthy man, and a reconditioning program for one who has been ill or injured. You should always consult your doctor about any aspect of your program which may require professional judgment. Throughout this book, we give clear precautions and suggestions about those aspects of physical fitness which deserve your physician's particular attention.

# 1

# PHYSICAL FITNESS— WHAT IT REALLY MEANS

Can you determine your physical condition by the number of pushups you can perform? Or by the ease with which you lift a 200-pound barbell over your head?

No.

Physical fitness cannot be measured in terms of strength, speed, endurance, or skill alone.

*True fitness can only be judged according to the individual man; by his physical ability related to his age, state of health, occupation, and history of exercise — as well as his daily living habits.*

As an example, a man of 25 may glide easily through 45 minutes of rigorous exercise every day — but on a comparative basis he may be in no better shape than a man of 45 whose limit of daily exercise is 15 minutes of mild calisthenics.

Dr. Lloyd Milburn, team physician for the San Francisco 49ers, says:

"True physical fitness is a *total concept*.

"It involves intelligent sleeping and working habits, intelligent play habits, and intelligent eating — as well as a sensible exercise program.

"As a result, being in fine physical condition means you are more efficient, not only bodily, but mentally."

## Learn Before You Leap

Don't flip impatiently through the pages of this book until you came to the actual exercise diagrams — because you'll just be cheating yourself.

A practical knowledge of your own body, and the basic principles of exercise which govern it, are as vital as the foundation of a building is to its structure. Physical fitness is a big subject, hence a little study is necessary to get the full benefit of the expert knowledge of the coaches, trainers, and doctors of the NFL.

Reading every page carefully is a worthwhile investment of time, for it will enable you to know exactly what you are doing — and why — every step of the way on the road to physical fitness.

## Three Common Misconceptions

Let's take the easiest way of learning what physical fitness is — by discovering first what it is *not*. We can do this by looking into three areas in which confusion and wrong ideas are common — and often harmful.

1 CONFUSING PHYSICAL FITNESS AND HEALTH    Do not confuse these two totally different concepts. *You can be healthy without being physically fit. But if you are physically fit, you must be healthy, too.*

The word "health," as generally used by doctors, means nothing more than freedom from disease or symptoms of dangerous bodily conditions. A tired, depressed, and over-worked businessman can be *healthy* even if he suffers from nervousness, bad digestion, and sleeplessness, and pants heavily if he so much as climbs two flights of stairs, so long as he doesn't have a disease or physical impairment.

If you don't feel energetic, optimistic, and rested, if getting out of bed in the morning is a chore and you drag through your day without inspiration, then a clean bill of health from your doctor should not be a source of cheer. But if you are physically fit, then you must be healthy. Your body has become a more efficient organism. You can perform more work at less bodily cost. You have better coordination, more endurance, strength, and even a healthier mental outlook.

2  BEWARE OF "MEASURING" PHYSICAL FITNESS  Many physical fitness programs offer charts, formulae, and tests of strength, speed, and endurance to help you determine your physical condition.

But remember these tests are based on average performance of large numbers of people. Your own performance deserves a *personal* evaluation in terms of your age, health, experience, and the length of time you have been exercising.

For instance, you may have increased from 20 to 50 the number of pushups you can perform. But this is only an indication of your arm and shoulder strength — not proof of strength in other muscle groups or of a generally improved condition.

"Every man, including the professional athlete, must base his training program on his *own needs*," says Roger McGill, trainer for the Pittsburgh Steelers.

"I don't mean in training camp, where conditioning is supervised, but during the off-season, where it's pretty much up to the men themselves to keep in shape.

"Ernie Stautner, our great tackle, doesn't have to concentrate on strength-building exercises, for he's a natural strong man whose 230 pounds are as hard as nails. He works to maintain flexibility and endurance, by playing a lot of handball.

"Another tackle, Ron Stehouwer, is also a 230-pounder, but works hard to build up his muscle size and strength because he realizes he hasn't yet developed to his full physical potential.

"These fine tackles are a perfect example of how two men can profit from different methods of training, even though both play the same role as athletes."

The tapemeasure can be just as misleading as a chart which claims to measure your progress. A program of exercise can add two inches of bulk to your biceps and taken an inch off your waistline. But your appearance is only a fraction of the picture of your health.

Perhaps you have exercised the wrong way for your natural body structure, and your small waist and thickened arms are actually unnatural — the product of intensive training that has created a marvelous appearance but has violated your natural body frame, symmetry, and ideal proportions.

"It would be foolish for Roger Brown, our 300-pound defensive tackle, to exercise for slimming purposes," says coach George Wilson of the Detroit Lions.

"His solid build and weight are what make him an effective blocker. A loss of 30 pounds might give him a more streamlined look and let him wear a smaller belt, but it would weaken him physically and impair his ability as an athlete."

Dale Messer, on the other hand, is a speedy, compact defensive back for the San Francisco 49ers. His forte is speed, his weapons flexibility and trickiness to match the feints of the pass receivers he must defend against. Ten pounds of additional weight on Dale's 175-pound frame would not measurably help him withstand the shock of constant impact. But it could slow him down a fraction of a second, and hinder his ability to cover opposing pass receivers.

So we see that "measuring" physical progress can be very misleading. Just as Roger and Dale differ radically in their body structures and skills, so do all men — even identical twins — differ, even if to a much lesser degree.

3 DON'T JUDGE STRENGTH, SPEED, AND ENDURANCE ON A COMPARATIVE BASIS These three physical attributes are vital to every athlete, and are greatly desired by most men. They are words that pack a wallop — but be careful. Each has its own meaning for you alone.

*Strength*, for example, has no simple definition. And football is the perfect sport to prove the point. A powerful 245-pound guard like Vince Promuto of the Washington Redskins may not be able to throw a football 30 yards. But a lean, 170-pound college quarterback, without half of Vince's brute strength, can easily arch a perfect spiral 60 yards through the air. Which of the two athletes is *stronger?*

And who is *faster:* a sprinter who can break ten seconds in the hundred-yard dash, or the miler who breaks four minutes in the mile?

And who has greater *endurance:* a swimmer who crosses the English Channel, or a calisthenics expert who can do 100 perfect pushups?

These questions are impossible to answer. Such words as strength, speed, and endurance must be defined not in terms of comparison to others, but in terms of the individual and the muscles he must call upon to perform his particular skill, whether he is an athlete or a tax expert.

## Personal Habits: The Basis of Physical Fitness

As a human being, you are the most nearly self-sufficient machine in the world. But the efficiency of your working parts — flesh, blood, bones, tissue, muscles, nerves, and organs — depends upon your treatment of them. Your daily living habits can build up or tear down the "machinery" of your body. Even if you are a young man with rippling muscles, raw strength, blazing speed, and catlike reflexes, you cannot remain in good condition if you drink and do not get proper sleep or nutrition three or four days a week.

Vince Lombardi, coach of the Green Bay Packers, knows his men regulate their own personal habits wisely.

"The true 'test of character' for my players comes during the off-season, when there is no supervision of their training, eating, or sleeping habits," says Vince.

"But every member of the Packers is a real professional. He knows that football is his livelihood — and that on any given play from scrimmage, the difference between a great player and an ordinary one is just half a step in speed or a fraction of a second in reflex action.

"My men are smart enough to put their physical conditioning ahead of everything else — by establishing and following good habits of diet, sleep, and exercise.

"When the bell rings for the start of a training season, I expect every one of them to report at or near peak condition.

"And I'm never disappointed."

Since the purpose of this book is to encourage and guide you, we do not feel it is our position to sermonize or regulate your personal habits. It is an accepted fact that the vast majority of American men use tobacco and alcohol as means of withstanding the pressures of the world and of their personal lives. But we urge every man to practice *moderation* in those personal habits which are clearly not in the best interest of his body.

## The Five Factors in Physical Fitness

We are now ready to look at the five basic ingredients which make up the "whole" of physical fitness.

Each of these parts is active rather than passive, for they require conscious effort and application on your part.

By recognizing all of these factors as being of equal importance, you will increase the benefits you receive from the time and energy you invest in any program of self-improvement.

1  SELF-DISCIPLINE    The effectiveness of any program of physical fitness depends upon how *consistently* you exercise.

If you *don't* want to improve yourself, if you think of exercising as an unpleasant chore rather than a pleasurable part of your day, then the odds are great you won't exercise on a regular basis. If so, it's your loss. We warn you that the benefits of occasional effort — exercising when you feel like it — will not be nearly as great as those of consistent performance, whether your program calls for activity three or seven days a week.

Exercising for twenty minutes daily, six days a week, a total of just two hours, is far more beneficial than exercising for two hours at a time twice a week, a total of four hours. In developing your body, your capacity for exercise must be built up gradually, and the only way to accomplish this is through consistent application. Your muscles cannot be toned by occasional spasmodic bursts of activity, for they will become fatigued rather than relaxed and sore rather than stimulated, and simply won't have the chance to build up the strength and resiliency necessary to take on more of a work load.

Concentrated activity cannot make up for "lost time." In this sense, exercise is like sleep. You can no more compensate for days of inactivity than you can make up for periods of insufficient rest by staying in bed 72 hours at a time. Our systems are not geared to such extremes, and we will pay the price in terms of bodily discomfort and depleted energy.

Your organs, which are stimulated so beneficially by regular exercise, can easily be strained by an overdose. Although the symptoms may not be readily apparent, especially to the young and strong, overexertion is simply flirting needlessly with disaster. Occasional but rigorous exercise is a shock to the body. A man who has not prepared himself gradually to withstand violent activity is subjecting himself to potential exhaustion or even serious illness, for he may be imposing a serious strain on his body.

"The danger of overexertion even applies to the professional athlete who gets out of shape during the off-season," says Tom Landry, coach of the Dallas Cowboys.

"The man who lets himself go, then has to fight his way back into condition, undergoes far more bodily strain than the man who keeps fit the year round.

"The years I've spent in the NFL as a player and coach have taught me that the players who never lose their edge of condition last far longer as athletes.

"That's why I encourage my men to keep in shape during the off-season — by testing them on the opening day of every training camp with the 'Landry Mile': Backs and ends must run a mile in under six minutes; linemen and linebackers in six and a half minutes. Anyone who fails to make the time limit will have to do a lot of extra running and calisthenics to get in shape.

"Knowing this helps 'inspire' the players to arrive in camp in top condition. So far, not one of them has failed the test."

*How To Attain Consistency*    Some men find it easier than others to exercise regularly. The athlete knows it's a matter of self-preservation. The artist, writer, or home-based salesman, who can choose his own hours of work and play, will have no problem finding time every day for physical activity. But the ordinary businessman, who leaves home early and returns in the evening, may feel more like having a drink and reading the newspaper than working out. He will find it easier to be consistent by following these suggestions:

First, try to choose a time of day or night when you will not be interrupted;

Second, chose a good location for your workouts where all the proper facilities as well as access to a hot shower and a change of clothes may be found;

Third, companionship may help inspire you. You can either exercise with members of your family or friends at home, or with a small group in a local gym. Not only will company make your exercise periods enjoyable socially as well as physically, but if one member of a group or family feels lazy that day, the others can prod him into activity.

Even under such ideal conditions, however, there will still be days when you just don't feel like exercising. This is when self-discipline becomes most important. You will find it helpful to remember the size of the goal you're striving for: A longer, healthier, and more enjoyable life.

2 EXERCISE Reaching a state of physical fitness without exercising is obviously impossible. But don't leap to the common and dangerous conclusion that activity alone guarantees attaining an improved condition.

Too many men suddenly become aware of their soft bodies and leap into a frantic physical training grind before they know what physical fitness is all about. They have a "love affair" with a set of weights or plunge into an advanced calisthenics program that would tax the strength of a professional football player. To make matters worse, they lack the perspective needed to tell the difference between improvement and bodily exhaustion; between aches caused by minor muscle stiffness and the danger signs of muscle strain.

The wrong kind of exercise — or too much exercise — can be dangerous. At the very least it is a waste of time, burning up precious energy and leaving you exhausted.

Dr. Francis Sweeny of the New York Giants offers this warning:

"*Caution* in exercising is vital — especially to men past 40 attempting to condition themselves after an extended period of inactivity.

"The greatest and most obvious danger is the risk of overtaxing your heart.

"In addition, muscles can be strained or torn. Even bones and joints can be damaged by too much stress.

"If you have an abdominal difficulty, such as a hernia, heavy exercises such as isometrics or weight training can make the condition much worse.

"Improper exercise often causes back injuries, due to incorrect positioning of the body while attempting to perform an exercise which requires great effort — such as lifting a heavy weight from the floor.

"The only intelligent approach to training — after having a thorough physical checkup, of course — is to follow consistently a planned program of physical fitness based on a *gradual increase of effort,* rather than an occasional urge to exercise."

By always remembering that exercise is just *one tool* to help you reach a peak of fitness, you will maintain the proper perspective, and avoid the danger of overexertion.

The selection of exercises for your program is of vital importance. In the chapter TAILOR YOUR PROGRAM TO YOUR OWN NEEDS and those that follow, you will receive complete and detailed guidance. First, the personal factors you must consider will be treated fully. Then the principles and purposes of each method of exercise — from calisthenics to isometrics — will be explained. Finally, each specific exercise will not only be discussed, but will be shown in simple diagrams.

**3 POSTURE** Many supposedly "complete" physical fitness programs forget all about posture. Other programs do mention the subject, but fail to recognize its importance.

*Good posture means more than good appearance: It is an active part of your fitness program.* Standing and walking properly are actually mild forms of exercise. For proper posture means that you are using your body frame and muscles in the manner in which nature intended — resulting in a minimum amount of strain on your body.

Even if you went completely without planned exercise, just standing, sitting, and walking correctly would guarantee you increased vitality.

*Poor posture is a threat to your health.* The vital organs in your body (heart, lungs, liver, spleen, kidneys, stomach, and intestines) depend upon having enough room to function properly, just as your arms and legs need room to work and play. If your body is bent the wrong way for an extended period, you are interfering with the natural functions of these organs, by cramping their room and freedom of action. Being hunched over not only prevents your organs from working properly, but also causes unnatural tension in your muscles, nerves, and ligaments. You feel generally fatigued, and so do your stomach and liver.

*Poor posture partially nullifies the benefits of your exercise program.* To a great degree, your vitality, suppleness, and feeling of well-being depend on how you walk, stand, and sit throughout the day. A vigorous workout may be a wonderful tonic, leaving you feeling fresh, vital, and full of energy. But if your body settles into an habitual slump minutes later, don't wonder why your energy is soon gone, and you feel "tired all over." Since poor posture puts your muscles under an unnatural strain for many hours every day, it is a direct cause of body fatigue.

"Not all posture problems are the result of laziness or bad habits," warns Dr. Theodore Fox of the Chicago Bears.

"In many cases, poor posture is caused by actual bone structure, or can be the result of an illness.

"I've seen unfortunate cases where a parent scolds his little boy or girl for having bad posture — not realizing it isn't the poor child's fault at all.

"In cases of bad posture which just don't seem to respond to an effort to stand and sit straighter, or where such effort is actually a strain on the body, a specialist should be consulted."

In the chapter POSTURE, you will see why poor posture so often is directly related to physical ills, especially in the case of older men. In addition, you will be shown the easiest methods of attaining — and maintaining — proper posture as a habit throughout the day.

4   NUTRITION   Unfortunately, many Americans eat a great deal but receive relatively little nourishment, for their appetites are determined by impulse and preference rather than according to a sensible dietary plan. A balanced diet is an absolute necessity. Food is your only means of replenishing the energy which your body constantly burns up. For the moment we are concerned with the word "diet" as it applies to one's normal eating habits — not to "dieting" for the purposes of weight control.

The two basic principles of proper diet are simple. First, check with your doctor to determine your ideal daily caloric intake. Secondly, your diet should be balanced to include the necessary amounts of proteins, carbohydrates, minerals, and vitamins.

Ed Block, the Baltimore Colts' trainer, comments on his team's eating habits:

"In training camp we give the players a carefully supervised diet of 4,000 calories a day — at least 1,000 calories more than the average man's daily intake.

"This would make most men fat, but the players burn up so much energy they remain physically firm.

"During the off-season, we talk to the married players' wives and suggest the type and amount of food to serve. The ladies are very cooperative in following our suggestions, and are a great help in keeping the men's weight down.

"Bachelors are a different story. We instruct them to eat well-balanced food, but we give nature a hand by supplying them with vitamin capsules, for many of them eat in restaurants, living on 'pick-up' meals rather than carefully choosing a balanced diet."

In the chapter WEIGHT CONTROL, we will discuss the subject of a balanced diet in more detail, and how to combine an intelligent diet with an exercise program to gain or lose weight.

5 SLEEP, REST, AND RELAXATION    The greatest athletes in the world couldn't possibly stay in top shape without enough sleep. There is simply no substitute for sleep, for it is man's basic source of recuperation, physically and psychologically.

Drugs, diet, will power, or even such an intensely emotional state as "being in love" may enable you to exist on three or four hours of sleep a night. But your body will eventually pay the price in terms of exhaustion, slower reflexes, and loss of endurance.

Medical books have offered different opinions as to how much sleep one needs, and college professors and scientists have argued their convictions for years. But there is no absolute authority on the subject. We believe that the amount of sleep you need is individual, and can best be determined by time and by trial and error. Once you discover your need, there is a simple, intelligent rule to follow: *Get the minimum amount of sleep you need consistently.*

If there is any change in your pattern, let it be additional sleep on weekends or holidays — but never settle for less than your minimum requirement. Taking short naps is an excellent practice when your schedule allows it, especially after vigorous physical exertion. For even 20 minutes of sleep will act as a tonic to help replenish your supply of energy.

If your body occasionally seems to "cry out" for extra sleep, by all means respect its demands. Your system may require the additional slumber to recover from overwork or mental strain, or to fight off anything from a common cold to a serious illness.

The related subjects of rest and relaxation will be discussed fully in the chapter SLEEP, REST, AND RELAXATION, where we will discuss the harm caused by lack of sleep and too much sleep, the nature of relaxation (including the need of vacations, or changes of scene, as a basic part of a healthy life), and the different types of fatigue — as well as their causes, dangers, and cures.

In Summary:     This chapter has defined the "philosophy" of physical fitness. We have tried to show you that it is a concept both physical and mental; that your own common sense must be a key factor in your program of physical improvement.

Further, we have pointed out the danger of relying too heavily on tests or charts to determine your condition. We have underscored the *absolute necessity* of having a complete physical examination before starting even the mildest of exercise programs.

The phrase "physically fit" describes a high level of health and bodily condition, attained by the sensible and consistent application of body-building exercises coordinated with the will to succeed, proper dietary procedures, good posture, and the necessary amount of sleep to balance your daily life.

# 2

# THE BENEFITS OF REGULAR
# EXERCISE

The man who has reached a high level of physical fitness
has a great deal in common with a racehorse. Once such an
animal is trained, his body becomes used to daily workouts.
If he isn't exercised regularly, he loses his fine edge of
speed and endurance. In addition, he becomes a nervous
bundle of frustrated energy.

In much the same manner, a well-trained man suffers if
he suddenly stops his accustomed program of exercise.

Not only would his high level of endurance, strength,
and flexibility diminish, but he would be liable to suffer
mental tension due to "unused energy."

Joe Kuharich, coach of the Philadelphia Eagles, gives another reason why it's a bad practice suddenly to stop
exercising:

"It's a lot easier to *keep* in shape than to *get* there," says
Joe.

"The man who stops training 'cold' is just making it
hard for himself. When the day comes that he gets dis-
gusted with his condition, he'll face the tough job of starting training all over again.

"Of course there are legitimate cases of a man having to

cut down on his training. An athlete, for instance, may suddenly be appointed a coach.

"But he shouldn't stop exercising. He should adjust by *gradually slackening* the intensity of his exercises over a period of several weeks, until he reaches a level of training best suited to his new living habits."

Consistent exercise encourages further activity. Once you are on the right road to physical fitness, nature aids your progress — by making you *desire* more of the energy-building and body-toning exercise that has lifted your entire system to a peak of efficiency. But increased energy, body tone, and endurance are not the only benefits of consistent exercise. There are many more.

## Healthier Muscles

Consistent exercise directly benefits your muscle *tone, endurance,* and *strength.*

IMPROVED MUSCLE TONE    *Muscle tone* is more than a neat phrase or vague description of a well-conditioned body. Technically, it is a healthy state of slight muscular contraction. In this condition muscles are not only more *efficient,* but also have far greater *flexibility.* They respond faster, use up less energy, and can work longer without fatigue than slack muscles.

An extreme but accurate example of someone whose muscles are "toneless" due to a lack of activity is the man who has been confined to bed for a long period. When he first gets out of bed and tries to walk, he feels weak all over, for his muscles have begun to wither, or atrophy. If one of his limbs has been in a cast, he finds that its muscles literally have shrunk in size.

It is a fact that well-toned muscles burn up 30 to 40 percent less energy in the performance of their daily work.

To ignore your muscles' need for exercise and expect to

have a responsive, supple body, is as impossible as denying a tree sunlight and water and expecting it to produce healthy branches.

GREATER MUSCLE STRENGTH    Strength is simply the ability to exert force by pushing, pulling, or lifting. Consistent exercise is the only way to develop strength, for sporadic activity only tires or strains muscles.

Strength is gained by *using muscles against some kind of an opposing force* — a form of exertion which makes muscles contract. The greater the contraction, the greater the muscle stimulation and development, both in strength and size.

A man with poor muscle tone and little strength is a good candidate for injuries. Sudden exertions — lifting, pulling, pushing, or even whirling around suddenly — can produce painful muscle strains and "pulls."

AVOIDANCE OF MUSCULAR TENSION    The fact that lack of proper exercise results in muscular "softness" or "flabbiness" has been pointed out by numerous newspaper and magazine articles, and has been harped on by everyone from physical education instructors to politicians. However, most so-called experts have failed to point out a danger every bit as great, but not nearly as obvious: the danger of muscular *tension*.

A man can see that he is soft and fat merely by looking in a mirror. But he cannot look beneath the surface and see the damaging effects of tension at work in his system. (Many of us are in the habit of assuming that *tension* refers to a mental state. But muscular tension is just as serious a problem.)

*Muscular tension* can best be illustrated by a simple comparison: When an animal is alarmed or excited it tenses, or flexes, almost all of its muscles. Then it either springs at the source of its fear or anger, or turns and runs away.

Either course of action rids the animal of its tension. When a man is alarmed or worried, his muscles tense in the same manner. But he rarely follows his healthy and instinctive reaction to fight or flee. As a result, the tension in his muscles remains — just as mental tension remains. This may be good for civilization, but it's hard on the man. (Certainly there is some merit in occasionally "blowing off steam.")

This sustained physical tension is a direct cause of bodily harm. It not only tightens muscles, but actually causes them to become physically shorter. If this process continues — and is not counteracted by exercise — the muscle gradually becomes "sick," and loses its shape, flexibility, and strength.

The danger of muscular tension varies with the individual. Men who constantly use their bodies vigorously, such as athletes, farmers, or laborers, have little to fear. But the man who sits behind his desk all day and then goes home and sits in front of a television set until bedtime had better watch out.

The cure for ordinary muscular tension is simple: Consistent exercise that vigorously stretches and flexes your muscles.

The following example makes this clear: In a clinic visited by thousands of people suffering from the common ailment of "lower back pain," doctors discovered that 75 percent of the complainers had no injury at all — just weakness or stiffness due to inactivity. The vast majority of them were healed by simple exercises that limbered, or stretched, their lower back muscles.

The same principle applies to *every part of your body:* Where there is a muscle, there is a need for exercise.

Dr. Erwin Mayer of the Baltimore Colts points out that not *all* cases of muscular tension can be blamed on physical inactivity:

"Some men just naturally have tight muscles in certain parts of their body," says Dr. Mayer.

"Our defensive end, Ordell Braase, suffers from chronic tight muscles of the lower back — despite the fact that he's always in top shape.

"To correct this condition, Ordell engages in a strenuous and consistent program of calisthenics which *stretch* his back muscles.

"This treatment helps keep his lower back muscles supple."

## Increased Efficiency of Body Organs

Besides better muscle tone and increased strength and endurance, there's another reason why you just plain "feel better" when your body is physically fit. Your internal organs have room to work as they should, uncramped by the weight of fat layers. You carry yourself with ease because well-conditioned muscles support your frame properly.

Dr. George Resta of the Washington Redskins comments:

"Your heart thrives on consistent activity — in that your 'cardiac reserve' is increased.

"In simple terms, this means that your heart profits from consistent exercise by growing stronger. As a result, whenever you exert strenuous physical effort, your heart has the 'reserve strength' to perform its functions without being overtaxed.

"In addition, consistent exercise helps both the digestive and respiratory systems work more effectively.

"And it helps improve your circulation and elimination of waste, by stimulating glands and body organs so that they perform their functions better."

The healthy, physically fit man is seldom plagued with indigestion, aches, pains, constipation, chronic fatigue, and all the other "minor" afflictions that rob a man of his feeling of well-being. Not so with the flabby-muscled man; he soon takes on a slumped appearance. (Ever notice how an erect carriage just seems to go naturally with a physically fit man?) No wonder. Supporting the body in its proper position takes strong, well-toned muscles. Without muscles, the whole body would sag.

Look closely at an NFL lineman. He may weigh anywhere from 220 to 300 pounds. Yet he doesn't sag, even though he may carry an extra "cushion" around his middle to help absorb the jarring impact of blocking and tackling. His magnificently conditioned muscles fully support his weight. Consistent exercise has made him truly physically fit. He looks well. He feels well. He is well — inside and out.

## Effective Weight Control*

A great deal of confusion exists about weight control, for, as in fashion, diet fads come and go — as do theories of intensive exercise programs for losing or gaining weight. There is only one sure, safe way to lose weight: Consistent exercise combined with a *reduced but balanced diet*.

Harland Svare, coach of the Los Angeles Rams, tells us how Rosey Grier, his star defensive tackle, lost over 20 pounds — without losing any strength:

"Rosey is an enormous man who'd shoot up to well over 300 pounds if he let himself go physically," says Harland.

"But he keeps in trim condition all the time.

"When he arrived at the Rams' training camp for his first season with the team, he cut 20 pounds off his weight, reducing from about 315 to 295.

"He did it by intelligent eating habits — by maintaining a well-balanced diet, but cutting way down on starches and sweets.

---

* This section does not apply to people with glandular disturbances or organic disorders. Their problems require medical attention.

"And in addition to his regular training routine, he did a tremendous amount of running and calisthenics.

"Since he combined a good diet with a sound exercise program, Rosey's weight reduction didn't cost him any loss of strength. And it added to his speed and mobility, for he still has the same big frame and the same strong muscles — with 20 less pounds to carry."

Just as there is only one good way to lose weight, there is but one sure, safe way to gain weight: consistent exercise combined with *an increased but balanced diet.*

Leo Murphy, trainer for the Cleveland Browns, tells us how tackle Dick Schafrath turned from an average-sized player into a really "big man":

"Dick reported to his first training camp weighing 218 pounds," says Leo.

"He wanted to put on solid weight, because he just wasn't big enough to block 250- and 260-pound defensive linemen.

"In just one year he did an amazing job of adding 40 pounds of muscle to his frame. His methods were simple.

"He followed a program of heavy weight training, which gradually increased his bulk, and did a lot of calisthenics and running which kept him hard and firm as he added the new weight.

"In addition, besides his regular diet he ate lots of steaks and malted milks. Now, at 258 pounds, he's one of the outstanding big linemen in the league — and he's still as hard as nails."

Even if your problem is so extreme that you want to lose or gain as much as 60 or 70 pounds, *do not take on a crash program involving either diet or exercise or both.*

Dr. John Best of the Pittsburgh Steelers comments:
"Losing weight too quickly can be a shock to your sys-

tem, depleting your energy and leaving you in a state of near exhaustion.

"Fatigue, in turn, makes you more susceptible to everything from a common cold to a serious illness.

"In addition, a crash diet may leave the body badly undernourished. The ill effects may not show for months or even years, but you may be risking your health tomorrow for a better appearance today.

"Losing weight naturally — and this means *gradually* — avoids placing a strain on your body, and in turn on your organs.

"Radically changing your normal diet and the method or degree of your normal exercise routine is flirting with danger."

In the chapter WEIGHT CONTROL, you will find a detailed discussion of the methods of losing and gaining weight by combining exercise and diet, and special exercise techniques for both purposes.

## A Better Mental State

Physical and mental fitness can never be truly separated, since one is related directly to the other. A physically conditioned man possesses an inner feeling of well-being. He has the confidence of knowing that no matter what his age, size, or stature, his "best foot is forward" both socially and in business. He feels full of energy and zest, eager to hop out of bed in the morning and attack his work for the day.

Our late President, John F. Kennedy, was a strong exponent of physical fitness. He hit the nail squarely on the head when he stated:

"The relation between the soundness of the body and the activities of the mind is subtle and complex. Intelligence and skill can function at their peak only when the body is healthy and strong."

Every action of the physically fit man exudes evidence of both inner and outer strength. "He looks like a success" is a phrase often applied to a man who stands straight and tall, walks with a positive stride, performs his daily work and play with vigor, and still has energy left to burn.

For the normally healthy man, burning up physical energy is an enjoyable pursuit. Investing his energy in a purposeful, positive direction gives him a genuine sense of satisfaction. At the same time it serves as a release which lessens mental tensions and helps him relax. The average man, in other words, will have better control over his emotions if he includes exercises or sports in his daily life.

But we must now issue a warning, to make sure you avoid a common and dangerous assumption:

*Although exercise does improve a man's mental state, it can never replace professional treatment for mental disorders — any more than it can heal physical ills.*

If your personal difficulties are so serious that they interfere with your leading a normal, well-balanced life, the solution to them might be provided by your doctor, psychiatrist, or minister.

Disturbed people should beware of throwing themselves into a physical fitness program for therapeutic purposes, because exercise can have a damaging effect upon them. For their mental condition may have caused abnormal changes in their body metabolism, energy balance, and basic body functions.

In Summary:   Exercise benefits the healthy man's mind and emotions. But it is not a method of overcoming mental problems.

## Protection Against Injury and Stress

The well-conditioned man can stand far more punishment

than his poorly conditioned brother. Many professional football players, for instance, withstand tremendous physical abuse from bigger, stronger men every Sunday during the NFL season.

Norm Van Brocklin, coach of the Minnesota Vikings, once played with Tommy McDonald, the speedy flanker back of the Dallas Cowboys. Norm is still amazed at Tommy's ability to take a beating:

"At 173 pounds, Tommy is one of the smallest men in the league," says Norm.

"And he constantly gets hit with tremendous impact by much bigger men — just a fraction of a second after he catches a pass.

"But he always bounces up and trots back into the huddle as if he hasn't even been tackled. Part of his toughness is mental, because Tommy is a magnificent competitor. But it can't be all mental, for a man with all the determination in the world couldn't take that kind of a beating unless he were in superb condition.

"I'm convinced the average young man of Tommy's age who took the same kind of punishment for just one game would end up in the hospital."

Bodily toughness, or fitness, cannot protect you from injuries resulting from events beyond your control, such as auto accidents. But the better conditioned a man's body is, the greater the chances of his recovering from a serious injury — and the quicker he will recover from minor physical damage.

Dr. Victor Ippolito of the Cleveland Browns comments:

"An athlete generally recovers from injuries more quickly than the average man.

"The fact that he usually receives immediate medical

treatment is one important reason why — but not the only reason.

"For the athlete is in better shape to embark upon a reconditioning program.

"Every portion of his body — not just his muscles — is physically fit and conditioned. His entire system 'cooperates' by working at maximum efficiency to speed his recovery."

Physical fitness is also a protection against fatigue. It gives a man the stamina, strength, and skill to carry on his daily routine at home, in the office, or in school without getting exhausted.

And it gives him something extra: *a margin of safety.* This "emergency reserve," which can only be developed through consistent exercise, is necessary to help you recover from emotional stress as well as physical damage.

An emotional blow — a death in the family, a divorce, even loss of a job — can have a devastating effect on health. A severe emotional shock can take an even greater toll on your body than depression, worry, or anger. The better your physical condition, the more reserve energy and confidence you will have to face and recover from misfortune of any kind — mental or physical.

# 3

## TAILOR YOUR PROGRAM TO YOUR OWN NEEDS

There is a great difference in training players in the National Football League and training the average man. The football player is always in good-to-excellent condition, even during the off-season. He is always a "young man," whether he is 20 or 35. He jumps right into a vigorous preseason training program without ill effects, and within a few weeks has built himself up to a magnificent peak of physical fitness.

A group of average men, on the other hand, varies all the way from the proverbial 98-pound weakling to a born "brute of a man." They are in vastly different states of bodily condition, and have widely varying capabilities of strength, speed, and endurance. As a result, their physical fitness programs must be very different.

In training 40 or more football players, NFL coaches and trainers carefully allow for the physical differences among them, and the different purposes for which they must train. A back or an end must emphasize speed. A guard or tackle must develop all his potential strength. But in the large sense of physical development, these differences are relatively minor, at least compared to a group of 40 men between the ages of 20 and 35 chosen at random.

In other words, members of a football team will go through essentially the same vigorous physical training grind, despite their individual differences. Each will be aiming at the same goals: toughness, absolute command of his body, an ability to withstand tremendous punishment, almost unbelievable endurance, and reflexes keyed to split-second reactions. Beyond this point, each player will concentrate on any *additional training* he needs to develop a particular ability or overcome a particular bodily weakness.

*Your* case is different from that of the professional football player. First, you must remember that, for the purposes of physical training, you are like no other man. The right physical fitness program for you must be highly individual, from the day you first start exercising.

Second, your program is *flexible,* and not a magic formula. If you fail to gain the benefits you desire, you must be willing to experiment intelligently, to try new methods of exercise, to make changes where and when necessary for your progress.

Trainer G. E. "Moose" Detty of the Philadelphia Eagles tells how center Jim Schrader derived great benefit by making a simple change in his training program:

"Jim has kept in top shape from the first day he became an Eagle," says Moose.

"But after six or seven years on the team, the 'spring' somehow seemed to leave his legs. He was still strong, but grew tired after running only a short distance.

"Then he cut down on strength-building exercises for his legs and began skipping rope. That one simple exercise made all the difference in the world.

"After just a couple of weeks of rope skipping, Jim's legs felt 'alive' again."

Third, your ego should not stand in your way. If you find you cannot comfortably handle as much of a work load as fast as a smaller, weaker appearing man, don't take it as a blow to your manhood. An intelligent physical fitness program must be tailored to your needs and abilities, not your pride.

Comparisons, it has often been said, are odious. In the world of physical fitness, they are at the very least useless, and can be dangerous. A program which turns one man into a superb physical specimen may badly overtax another's body and leave him exhausted.

Therefore, before deciding upon your own program, you should carefully consider a number of important personal factors.

## Your Age Is an Important Factor

There are no exact rules which tell you what you can or cannot do at a certain age. But *everyone* must build up to a peak condition carefully and gradually.

Up to the age of 30, most normally healthy men can take on an intensive training program without risk of bodily harm.

At 35, a man should think twice, even three times, about launching himself into an intensive training grind. At this age he is still young and active and at a wonderful peak of both physical and mental maturity. But there is little likelihood of his becoming a professional athlete or suddenly embarking upon a career which calls for strenuous physical effort.

With rare exceptions, the man of 35 who is genuinely interested in being physically fit should get everything he needs from a moderate schedule of exercise. This will not only develop his body to a satisfactory degree, but will also leave him with enough strength for such sports as golf, bowling, or tennis. To launch himself into a more vigorous program would, we think, require a most unusual set of circumstances.

We see no reason why a man at the age of 40 or over should need anything more than a moderate exercise program. Even if he starts out in poor condition, such a program will not only assure him of reaching a highly satisfactory physical level, but will keep him there. His entire body will be toned and he'll have enough energy remaining to engage in recreational sports.

The man of 50 and over can follow the same general program, but he should perform fewer exercises. *He should never exercise to the point of exhaustion.* There is no reason why most men of 65 can't swim, play golf, or bowl. Most men of 75, who have kept physically fit, can still swim and take walks — even play golf and bowl — if they don't overexert themselves.

Dr. James Nixon of the Philadelphia Eagles offers the following advice to senior citizens:

"You must remember that the older you become, the more subject you are to strain or fatigue.

"But older men should make mild exercise a daily habit, for it will keep them from slipping into a level of general physical incapacity.

"Too many old people drop dead as the result of having to make a sudden effort — such as shoveling their way out of a snowstorm or pushing a stalled car. The reason is simple: Their hearts and bodies have gone so long without stimulating activity that they have built up no 'reserve energy' for an emergency.

"Exercise for older men can take several forms. Mild calisthenics are very beneficial. Swimming and walking are ideal, since they can be performed slowly and with little exertion.

"Even the healthy man of 90 will benefit from some mild exercise every day."

## Your Health Must Be Carefully Evaluated

We repeat the principle we stated so strongly earlier in the book: *If you have physical difficulties, illness, or handicaps of any nature, do not expect exercise to correct the trouble. See a doctor or a specialist.*

If you are in good health, but have a history of serious illness involving heart trouble, high blood pressure, or a serious disease, then the rule you must follow is simple: *Check with your doctor first, then proceed slowly and care-*

*fully on the road to physical fitness under his continuing counsel.*

If you are young, and your malady disappears with time and proper living habits, then in all probability your doctor will let you progress to a more intensive level of exercise. But this is highly individual, just as the effects of disease are individual. Your doctor is the only man to give you competent advice.

Dr. James Nellen of the Green Bay Packers comments:

"There is a great difference between a physical fitness program and a reconditioning program.

"A man who is recovering from an injury or illness must work hand in hand with a doctor. In addition, he must realize the necessity of taking plenty of time to build up his strength and endurance — much more time than a healthy man of the same age would need.

"Too much exercise for a man with a weakened body can act as a poison to his system. Impatience and bad judgment which make him 'bite off more than he can chew' can put him right back into a sickbed."

For older men with chronic physical problems which deplete their supply of energy, there are mild forms of exercise which hardly take any effort: practicing good posture, stimulating the whole body by "stretching" arms, legs, and trunk as one does while yawning, and taking slow, short walks. These are safe, mild tonics for muscles and organs, even for most men just out of the hospital.

In Summary:  Common sense coupled with competent medical advice will answer any questions concerning a safe physical fitness program for you.

## How Your Occupation and History of Exercise Are Related

As we have discussed, suddenly embarking upon a strenuous program of exercise is a shock to your system. The only way to avoid this shock is to become physically fit *gradually*. It is always far wiser and safer to proceed too slowly than too quickly.

Your occupation and history of exercise are, in most cases, directly related. A traveling salesman or mailman, who moves about on his feet every day, will not have much trouble adjusting to a regular program of exercise, and a reasonable calisthenics program should be no strain for his system. After three or four weeks of practice, he can then start a more intensive program.

But an executive, who has sat at a desk for ten years and whose greatest physical accomplishment has been lifting his third martini with a steady hand, must use caution. He must start with light workouts, build up the number of exercise repetitions very carefully, and be extremely careful to stop short of fatigue. For he must avoid damaging tense, unused muscles or putting too great a strain on a "rusty" body system that has gone for many years without the proper physical stimulation.

## How Your Body Type Determines Your Capacity

The right physical fitness program for you also must take into account your *body type*. Contrary to popular notions, this involves far more than height and weight. It concerns your overall body structure: the width of your frame, the size of your bones, the thickness and quality of your muscles.

Three people of identical height may have three entirely different body types — and thus have completely different needs in terms of bodily conditioning.

To illustrate the point, let's take three players from the National Football League — Jerry Kramer, Greg Larson, and R. C. Owens. Each man is exactly 6 feet, 3 inches tall, and each is an excellent example of the three classic body types: *mesomorph, endomorph,* and *ectomorph.*

Jerry Kramer, a 250-pound offensive guard for the Green Bay Packers, is a perfect specimen of the *mesomorph.* He is built heavily and squarely; he is large-boned, heavy-muscled, thick-necked, strong, and solid.

Carl Jorgensen, the Packers' trainer, analyzes Jerry:

"Although he is physically 'thick,' Jerry is so well-rounded an athlete he doesn't have to emphasize any particular phase of his training.

"Blessed with excellent speed for a big man, he exercises to maintain his muscularity and keep his body firm. In addition, he runs to keep his speed, and practices calisthenics for endurance and agility.

"Even though he is an extreme body type, Jerry's build is perfect for an offensive guard. For he needs his bulk and raw power to block opposing defensive linemen who are usually the heaviest players in the league."

An *endomorph,* like center Greg Larson of the New York Giants, is also large, big-boned and heavily muscled at 250 pounds. But where Kramer is "square," Larson is "round." His huge body tends to excess weight, and unless he keeps in top condition, he can put on fat in a hurry, with a resulting loss in speed, mobility and supply of energy.

Says Allie Sherman, coach of the Giants:

"Greg is an outstanding young center with tremendous natural strength.

"But because of his body structure, he has to be careful not to put on excess weight. Although he works to maintain his strength, he must put particular emphasis on calisthenics, running, and playing handball the whole year round — to make sure he stays hard and agile.

"Greg is such a willing worker his body stays firm and well-toned despite his size."

R. C. Owens, a 195-pound offensive end for the New York Giants, is a healthy prototype of the *ectomorph*. He is tall and lean with a relatively light body frame and small bones. His muscles are long rather than thick and bulky. He is clearly built for speed and flexibility rather than for raw strength.

Don Shula, R. C.'s former coach at Balitmore, comments:

"R. C. would be making a big mistake trying to become a strong man by adding bulk or muscle to his frame. His shiftiness and ability to leap high into the air for passes depend upon his supple, 'loose' body.

"He keeps his skills at peak sharpness by maintaining a fine edge of conditioning the year round — constantly emphasizing speed, endurance, and agility."

It is important that you realize only about two out of every ten of us — whether football players or average men — have definite body types like Kramer, Larson, and Owens. *The vast majority of men are somewhere between two types, with physical characteristics of each.*

Every player in the NFL has a special and particular job to perform. As a result, *each player works to develop those abilities dictated by his body type.* If a player falls *between* two types, he will try to develop the best characteristics of each. Jim Gibbons, a 220-pound offensive end for the Detroit Lions, is a perfect "in-between." He has characteristics of both the ectomorph (tall and slender) and the mesomorph (square and powerful). Like R. C. Owens, his role as a pass receiver necessitates his concentrating on speed and endurance so he can outrun would-be tacklers. But at the same height of 6 feet, 3 inches, his extra 25 pounds let him bowl over enemy defenders as well.

DO NOT EMPHASIZE BODILY EXTREMES    If you happen to be one of the three classic body types, you should not attempt to make big muscles bigger or keep a slim body as hard as nails — unless you have a specific reason for doing so.

Instead, you should aim at "styling" your body toward "average build," by losing weight if you are heavy and gaining if you are thin.

The average working man built like Jerry Kramer has a natural tendency to put on weight because of his heavy body structure. Should he try to exercise for larger, stronger muscles the way Jerry does? No. The mesomorph not involved in a violent contact sport should exercise to keep his weight down while remaining firm and supple. This brings his heavy, solid frame closer to an average body build, which combines muscularity and hardness with symmetry, flexibility, and speed.

How about the non-athlete built like Greg Larson? He too would be foolish to try and maintain bulk, for he doesn't need Greg's muscular "cushioning" against impact from opposing players. The endomorph's aim should be like that of the mesomorph: to slim down as much as possible, to develop speed and flexibility.

And how about the busy executive built with the "string bean" type of build? The same common-sense principle applies: with the "average body build" in mind, he should exercise both to gain suppleness and to add more muscle.

In other words, you should *compensate for,* rather than add to, any over- or underdeveloped body structure. Extremes of strength, bulk, or speed will serve no useful purpose in making sales calls or designing bridges.

## Beware of False Values

Pity the poor man who believes the chart on a drugstore scale telling him he should weight exactly 178 pounds because he's six feet tall.

Other so-called indexes of physical fitness are just as inaccurate. They "advise" us as to how many pushups a man of 30 should be able to perform, but fail to consider that such a man may be a a physical laborer who can barely do 10 repetitions, or a top-flight golfer who can manage 30 repetitions only at the price of temporary exhaustion.

They advise us how much weight a man of 200 pounds should be able to lift above his head. But they fail to consider the fact that he may be a 6-foot, 10-inch basketball player with little strength for lifting bulk, or a squat, muscular stevedore who can almost lift a horse.

Another common type of "accomplishment index" is a statement such as, "A high school senior should be able to run the hundred yard dash in 12.8 seconds."

One high school senior may be skinny, undernourished, ill-coordinated, and a terrible athlete. However, he somehow manages to race across the finish line in the required time before flopping on his face from exhaustion. His schoolmate may be stronger, healthier, beautifully proportioned, and an excellent all-around athlete who is just not a fast runner. He may cross the finish line a tenth of a second later, but he is hardly breathing hard from the effort.

It is obvious that the "12.8 second" factor is absurd; that a physically inferior boy is judged "better" than a clearly superior athlete, because of one-tenth of a second on a stop watch. Such a "judgment" considers only the factor of speed — and even that only over a limited course — and ignores such vital factors as condition, size, strength, general athletic ability, coordination, and endurance.

So remember that the tapemeasure and the stop watch only consider one dimension of a man's true ability and condition.

By considering your own state of health, age, occupation, and history of exercise, as well as your body structure, you will be able to set up realistic training goals for yourself, and can sensibly judge your progress on the road to becoming physically fit.

# 4

# THE DIFFERENT TYPES
# OF EXERCISE

As we have stated in a dozen ways throughout this book, we do not believe there is such a thing as a single "perfect program" of physical fitness based upon a standard routine or a specific group of exercises.

As a result, we have set up *three basic programs*. Not only does each vary in intensity, but each is flexible. No matter what your age or condition, you can "custom build" a program to fit your own ambitions, and your own body.

First, let's take a look at the different forms of exercise which make up the three programs:

Although there are many forms of exercise — including sports, walking, running, and even practicing good posture — the three principal or most common forms of exercise are calisthenics, isometrics, and weight training.

## Calisthenics

Calisthenics always involve *movement*. They build *tone, endurance, flexibility,* and *strength.*

Every coach, doctor, and trainer in the NFL recognizes the absolute necessity of calisthenics in the training program of his players.

George Halas, coach of the Chicago Bears, says:

"Calisthenics are the very foundation of our team's training program. Not only do they help the players maintain agility, coordination, and quick reflexes, but they keep their muscles *stretched*, or loose.

"This enables even our most muscular players to build tremendous strength by performing heavy weight training and isometrics — exercises which by themselves might tend to shorten and tighten muscles — without ill effects.

"There is no substitute for calisthenics — for anyone. They are just as vital to the man of 70 who follows the mildest of physical conditioning programs, as to the young, tough, and capable professional athlete."

## Weight Training

The principle involved is simple: Specific muscles are flexed against a strong opposing force.

Weight training involves *movement:* The pitting of your strength to push, pull, or lift a certain number of pounds which you can gradually increase as you grow stronger.

This causes great muscle stimulation, forcing muscles to grow in both *size* and *strength*. This is why weight training is often referred to as the "body-building" exercise.

Since weight training involves repetitions, a great deal of energy must be exerted. Therefore, *weight training should be practiced only every OTHER day.*

## Isometrics

Isometrics are simply pushing, pulling, or lifting against an *immovable object*—by exerting *maximum* force for a few seconds. The "object" can be part of your own body or something stationary such as a metal bar, a wall, or doorway.

*Isometrics can be practiced EVERY day.*

## Differences Between Weight Training and Isometrics

All too often these two forms of exercise are compared as being equal in principle, value, and result, in that they are both simply "strength-building" exercises, and the choice of one over the other is no more than a personal preference.

Nothing could be further from the truth. Granted, both methods of exercise do build strength. *But there are differences in both their purposes and results.*

ISOMETRICS firm and strengthen muscles more rapidly with less effort.

They make little contribution to endurance. *Therefore, isometrics can never constitute a complete exercise program, but must be combined with calisthenics.*

WEIGHT TRAINING leads to *increased muscle size.*

Since the movement involved takes your muscles through a full range of action again and again (by repetitions), weight training builds *tone* and *endurance* as well as strength.

ISOMETRICS cannot be measured without the use of special equipment.

WEIGHT TRAINING *can* be measured, in terms of both the exact number of pounds a man lifts during any given exercise and the number of repetitions he performs.

Different combinations of weights and repetitions produce different kinds of benefits. We can see this clearly by considering three possible weight-training programs:

A heavy weight used with relatively few repetitions would roughly approximate the results of isometrics: Since there is little movement and great muscle-flexing, the accent is clearly on *strength-building* rather than endurance;

Using a moderate weight with a moderate number of repetitions puts an equal emphasis on *strength and endurance;*

A very light weight used with many repetitions would almost approach calisthenics: It will produce greatly increased *endurance,* but will cause little increase in strength.

In other words, weight training can be adjusted from one extreme of being a strength-builder (like isometrics) to the other extreme of building tone and endurance (like calisthenics).

The formula is simple:

More weight with less repetitions equals *strength;*

Less weight with more repetitions equals *tone and endurance.*

*Warning:* Young men often make the unfortunate mistake of building huge muscles by using heavy weights with few repetitions — without balancing their exercises by practicing calisthenics.

Such huge muscles are in danger of becoming shortened — or "bound." In this state, you may have great strength, but only limited flexibility. Being "muscle-bound" prevents a high level of athletic ability.

Since ISOMETRICS require the application of your full strength, they cannot be used to recondition weakened or damaged limbs or muscles.

WEIGHT TRAINING, on the other hand, can be used to *rehabilitate* an injured or weakened muscle — for the simple reason that you can start with a very light weight and gradually increase it over a period of time.

*(Warning:* Do not attempt to use weights to overcome the results of an injury or illness *without specific instructions from a doctor.)*

Dr. Richard Thompson, team physician for the Detroit Lions, offers a perfect example of the use of weights on the basis of progressive resistance to rehabilitate a player with a serious injury:

"Joe Schmidt, our fine linebacker, suffered a dislocated shoulder," said Dr. Thompson.

"We waited about six weeks after his operation, then began a program using very light weights of no more than five pounds. Joe picked up the small weights in his hand and moved his arm around in all possible positions, performing basic shoulder exercises with a great number of repetitions.

"This not only restored flexibility, but added a little strength.

"As the shoulder got better and better, we gradually added more and more weight; in other words, *progressively adding more resistance.*

"Finally Joe was able to do all the shoulder exercises easily while holding 20 to 25 pounds in his hand. Not only had his shoulder regained its full flexibility, but it was as strong as ever.

"Joe was then able to practice weight training and isometrics just the way he did before his injury."

In Summary:   Here are the "pros and cons" of isometrics and weight training, which are of great importance to men who choose between the two:

| ISOMETRICS | WEIGHT TRAINING |
| --- | --- |
| The *quickest* builder of raw strength; | Increases strength; |
| Exercises can be done *every day;* | Exercises should only be done *every other day;* |
| *Little or no equipment needed;* equipment is relatively inexpensive; | Complete training program requires *considerable equipment or access to a gym;* |
| Requires *little time,* with only short rests between exercises; | Can be quite *time-consuming,* requiring moderate rests between exercises; |
| Can be performed *in privacy* of room or office, without having to change from street clothes; | Must exercise *where weights are located;* changing into old clothes necessary since workout produces |

Limited increase in muscle size;

Exercise muscle *in one position* only;

*Cannot constitute a complete workout;* must be combined with calisthenics;

Increase in your strength must be measured by periodically lifting weights or using special testing equipment.

perspiration;

Greater increase in muscle size;

Exercises muscles through *complete range of movement;*

*Can constitute a complete workout* (if you use light weights with many repetitions);

Can measure developed strength on a pound-by-pound basis.

*The three forms of exercise are divided into three levels:* In the chapters CALISTHENICS, WEIGHT TRAINING, and ISOMETRICS, each form of exercise is divided into three levels: BASIC, ADVANCED, and INTENSIVE. This assures you of *maximum flexibility* in constructing your program. (Do not confuse these levels with the three programs themselves. It is perfectly possible to use a BASIC group of exercises, for instance, in Program II, as you will soon see.)

*Exercises are also divided into muscle groups:* In the same chapters, you'll see that each exercise is classified according to *basic muscle groups of the body,* such as back, abdominal, and leg muscles. This is to give you a sound basis for planning your program. It will help you choose a combination of exercises which will stimulate and tone your entire body. In addition, it will help you choose exercises to emphasize development of certain body areas.

Incidentally, an exercise specifically designed to benefit one muscle group actually will be helpful to others as well. For example, pushups primarily benefit the arms and shoulders, but they also develop the stomach and back. (If you don't believe it, feel someone's stomach when he is doing pushups.)

Now let's take a look at the three basic programs.

# 5

## THE THREE BASIC PROGRAMS

### PROGRAM I — For the Average Man

| | |
|---|---|
| **Its Purpose** | To maintain a good level of body tone, endurance, and coordination without emphasizing development of strength.<br>It should take from 10 to 20 minutes a day. |
| **For Whom** | The "average man" who wants to develop and maintain a well-conditioned body — with a minimum amount of time and effort. |
| **What It Is** | First, *warm-up calisthenics;*<br>Followed by either *BASIC* or *ADVANCED calisthenics.* |
| **Its Flexibility** | If you desire a very mild program, simply perform the seven exercises which make up the BASIC group of calisthenics.<br>If you want a more strenuous workout, either add more repetitions |

or new exercises, or progress to the
ADVANCED group of ten calisthenics.

|  |  | Page |
|---|---|---|
| **Where To Find It** | WARM-UP calisthenics | 64-67 |
| | BASIC calisthenics | 54-55 |
| | ADVANCED calisthenics | 55-56 |

## PROGRAM II — For the Working Man

**Its Purpose**  To develop an improved level of strength, as well as tone and endurance.

It should take between 15 and 45 minutes a day.

**For Whom**  The man who wants more than Program I offers. It will have special appeal for the man who wants to improve his skill in certain sports, such as golf, bowling, or tennis; the man who has generally underdeveloped muscular structure; or the man with a particular bodily weakness he wants to improve.

**What It Is**  First, *warm-up calisthenics;*
Followed by *calisthenics* as in Program I;
Then a choice of *weight training* or *isometrics* or *both*.

Optional: *Special exercises* for developing particular muscles.

**Its Flexibility**  If you choose *both* weight training and isometrics, you have no decision to make. But making a choice between them will require some thought.

HOW TO CHOOSE BETWEEN WEIGHT TRAINING AND ISOMETRICS
First, consider the summary of their advantages and differences on pages 44-45.

Two common-sense considerations are offered by Jack Christiansen, coach of the San Francisco 49ers:

"Appearance is one big factor," says Jack.

"A scrawny-looking individual might prefer weight training — for it builds greater muscle size than isometrics.

"A heavy man, on the other hand, might do better to choose isometrics — which strengthens without adding bulk.

"Time is also important. Where one man might have time for weight training, the busy executive would probably prefer isometrics — because it requires far less time and he can have a complete workout in the privacy of his office."

In Summary:    You must consider all the personal factors such as age, health, the amount of time you are willing to invest, and your body build, as well as your personal goals in terms of endurance, strength, and appearance.

The following chart outlines the possible combinations of calisthenics, weight training, and isometrics under Program II. (Remember that in the chapters CALISTHENICS, WEIGHT TRAINING, and ISOMETRICS the exercises are divided into three groups: BASIC, ADVANCED, and INTENSIVE.)

| Choice number | Calisthenics | Weight Training | Isometrics |
|---|---|---|---|
| 1 | BASIC | BASIC OR ADVANCED | |
| 2 | ADVANCED | | BASIC OR ADVANCED |
| 3 | BASIC | BASIC | BASIC |
| 4 | INTENSIVE | | |

*Following this chart is very simple:*

**Choice #1:** If you have chosen *weight training,* you can see that you need only perform BASIC calisthenics.

*Why:* Weight training tones as well as strengthens, therefore there is need for gaining endurance and flexibility through calisthenics.

**Choice #2:** If you have chosen *isometrics,* you can see that you should perform ADVANCED calisthenics.

*Why:* Isometrics develop great strength, some body tone, but little endurance; thus calisthenics, as the only source of endurance, must be emphasized.

**Choice #3:** If you have chosen both *weight training* and *isometrics,* we suggest you limit them both to BASIC — and do the same with *calisthenics.*

*Why:* Such a program offers an excellent balance in terms of tone, strength, and endurance.
(If you desire a more strenuous exercise routine, we suggest that you consider Program III.)

**Choice #4:** If you have chosen INTENSIVE calisthenics alone, you can use Program I as a basis, and add new exercises and more repetitions, as well as special exercises, in order to design a program to fit your needs perfectly.

*Note:* Calisthenics alone will not offer the strength-building benefits included in the three other choices. Therefore we recommend it only for people who want to develop tremendous agility, endurance, and flexibility.

## Special Exercises

Program II also offers special exercises for two specific purposes:

1  *To develop muscle groups used in each popular sport,*
so you can become a better athlete.

2  *To develop weak muscles or weak body areas.*

## Sports Can Be a Part of Program II

If you are actively athletic, you should make allowances in
your program for sports, since your exercises must relate
to your daily life on a common-sense basis.

If one day you play 18 holes of golf, there is no need to
perform leg exercises. If you spend an afternoon on the
tennis or handball court, your "calisthenics" for the day
have been done.

## Where To Find Program II

|  | Page |
|---|---|
| WARM-UP calisthenics | 64-67 |
| BASIC calisthenics | 54-55 |
| ADVANCED calisthenics | 55-56 |
| BASIC weight-training | 105-6 |
| ADVANCED weight-training | 106-7 |
| BASIC isometrics | 137 |
| ADVANCED isometrics | 138 |
| SPECIAL exercises | 61, 96-103, 157-60 |

# PROGRAM III—
## For Physical Fitness "Bugs"

Its Purpose     To build a *very high level* of strength,
                flexibility, endurance, and tone, as well as
                to develop muscle size and improved
                appearance.

                There is no "average" time requirement,
                as this program varies greatly with the
                individual.

**For Whom**     The man who wants to reach a superb level of physical fitness, such as the aspiring professional athlete or the man really dedicated to bodily conditioning — the physical fitness "bug."

(*Warning:* Unless you want to develop endurance, tone *and* strength to a high degree, *and* bigger muscle size, Program II may be better suited to your needs. Program III is recommended only for the physically hardy, who wish to condition themselves on a level with that of the professional athlete.)

**What It Is**     First, *warm-up calisthenics.*
Then *calisthenics* AND *weight training* AND *isometrics.*
Optional: *Special intensive exercises* such as wind sprints and rope climbing.

**Its Flexibility**     The following chart offers four choices. Any one offers a well-balanced program in terms of tone, strengthening, endurance, and flexibility.

| *Choice number* | *Calisthenics* | *Weight Training* | *Isometrics* |
|---|---|---|---|
| 1 | ADVANCED | ADVANCED | ADVANCED |
| 2 | ADVANCED | INTENSIVE | ADVANCED |
| 3 | INTENSIVE | ADVANCED | INTENSIVE |
| 4 | INTENSIVE | INTENSIVE | INTENSIVE |

Jack Rockwell, trainer for the St. Louis Cardinals, explains the merits of this intensive program in simple terms:

"CALISTHENICS are a vital part of every man's exercise program, since every joint structure and muscle group should be taken through a *complete range of movement* at least twice a week to avoid tightness and maintain tone.

"ISOMETRICS offers the best method of quickly building that *raw strength* which supplies the 'explosive power' used by professional athletes.

"WEIGHT TRAINING offers both *strength* and *endurance,* and also develops bulk and size. This not only creates an improved appearance, but enables you literally to become a bigger man.

"This program is basically that used by many NFL players. In addition, they all do a great deal of running, which is such a vital part of football, and for which there is no substitute."

## Where To Find Program III

# REVIEW OF EXERCISE BENEFITS

Before going into the details of exercises in the following chapters, let's look at a very simple table. This table summarizes the comparative benefits of each type of exercise — how much it contributes to building muscle tone, endurance, bulk and size, and strength. This table will be helpful in planning your program.

| | CALISTHENICS | | WEIGHT TRAINING | | | ISOMET-RICS |
| | Basic or Advanced Level | Intensive Level | Light Weights Many Repetitions | Moderate Weights Moderate Number of Repetitions | Heavy Weights Few Repetitions | |
|---|---|---|---|---|---|---|
| MUSCLE TONE | 1 | 1 | 1 | 1 | 2 | 2 |
| ENDURANCE | 2 | 1 | 2 | 2 | 3 | 3 |
| BULK AND SIZE | 4 | 3 | 3 | 1 | 2 | 3 |
| STRENGTH | 4 | 3 | 3 | 2 | 1 | 1 |

KEY

1 — Excellent
2 — Good to Excellent
3 — Fair
4 — Little or None

# 6

## CALISTHENICS

Calisthenics should be part of every physical fitness program, and should be performed every day you exercise. For the sake of simplicity, we offer three fundamental groups of exercises:

BASIC:         7 mild exercises
ADVANCED:   10 vigorous exercises
INTENSIVE:  Any number of vigorous exercises plus special exercises

### The BASIC Group

These include a minimum of seven mild exercises — a warm-up exercise and one for each major muscle group. We suggest the following basic exercises which we describe in detail later in this chapter.
Important:    Before you perform any exercise be sure to read the next section of this chapter: "How To Perform Calisthenics."

*Page*

(1)  5 to 10 Jumping Jacks (warm-up to benefit all body muscles)                              64

(2)   5 to 10 Deep Knee Bends (leg muscles)          89

(3)   5 to 10 Side Stretchers (lateral trunk
        muscles)                                                      73-74

(4)   5 to 10 Toe Touchers (back muscles)          78-79

(5)   3 to 6 Neck Flexes (neck muscles)            94-95

(6)   5 to 10 Leg-ups  (abdominal muscles)            83

(7)   5 to 10 Pushups (chest, arm, and shoulder
        muscles)                                                         68

## The ADVANCED Group

You can incorporate advanced calisthenics in your physical fitness program in one of two ways:

1   Perform more repetitions of basic exercises.
2   Select more difficult or "advanced" exercises instead of basic exercises.

For (1) above, we suggest 10 to 20 repetitions of each exercise.

For (2), which will probably interest more people, we suggest the series of ten advanced exercises listed below. Taken together, these exercises constitute a rigorous, even a violent program of calisthenics, depending on the number of repetitions you perform and how much energy you throw into exercising.

                                                                    *Page*

(1)   1 minute or 30 repetitions, Running in
        Place (warm-up to benefit all body muscles)   65

(2)   5-8 Bar Hangs (warm-up to benefit all
        body muscles)                                               66-67
        *or:* 1 minute of Shadow Boxing for the
        same benefits                                                  65

(3)   15 to 20 Side Stretchers (lateral trunk
        muscles)                                                      73-74

(4)   15 to 20 Back Stretchers (back muscles)     80-81

(5) 15 to 20 Squat Jumps (leg muscles)     91

(6) 6 to 12 Leg Splits (abdominal muscles)   86-87

(7) 15 to 20 Side Benders (lateral trunk muscles)     76

(8) 10 to 15 Wrestler's Bridge (neck muscles)     95

(9) 10 to 20 Sit-ups (abdominal muscles)   85-86

(10) 15 to 20 Squat Thrusts (chest, arm, and shoulder muscles)     70

## The INTENSIVE Group

You can construct an INTENSIVE calisthenics program in one of three ways:

1  Perform more repetitions of advanced exercises.

2  Perform additional advanced exercises to benefit any muscles which need special work.

3  Add "special" exercises such as road work, etc.

It is just about impossible to be specific about INTENSIVE calisthenics. We believe that the group of 10 advanced exercises, using 25 to 40 repetitions of each, offers an excellent intensive program.

We have also included *special calisthenics:* miscellaneous exercises which are all highly intensive.

## How To Perform Calisthenics

As easy as calisthenics may appear, there is a right way and a wrong way to do them. If you expect to derive the full benefits of each exercise, observe each of the following rules.

FOLLOW DIRECTIONS EXACTLY   Under each exercise in the next section of this chapter, you will find *complete directions and diagrams* showing you exactly how to perform the proper movements. Some of the movements may not seem easy or "natural" at first, but don't let that prevent you from sticking to directions. Before too long your muscles will respond and you will be able to perform each exercise easily.

ALWAYS WARM UP BEFORE PERFORMING OTHER CALISTHENICS
If you don't, you run the risk of muscle strain.

Ed Rozy, trainer of the Chicago Bears, says:

"One of the most important things I drill into rookies' heads is, *always* warm up before calisthenics, and *always* practice calisthenics before engaging in more violent exercise. This applies to the football field, to the isometric power rack, a weight-training session, or even to a man throwing a football through a rubber tire in his back yard.

"Starting strenuous exercise with a 'cold' body is dangerous, for you can easily rip a muscle and be out of action for a week or more.

"For anything more than a mild program of calisthenics, I suggest a minimum period of five minutes of leisurely warming up."

DON'T FORCE YOUR MUSCLES BEYOND THEIR ABILITIES  In the Toe Toucher exercise, for example, you may not be able to touch your toes right away. And it may be several weeks before you can. But be patient. Bend only as far as you comfortably can. With constant practice, you will become more flexible.

If you should foolishly force your muscles beyond their capabilities and lunge down at your toes, the torn back or leg muscle that may result will prevent you not only from touching your toes, but from doing any kind of stretching, for weeks or even months.

BREATHE NORMALLY DURING EXERCISES  Failure to breathe freely interferes with the purpose of conditioning. When you exercise, your body starts to use up energy at a much faster rate than usual. As a result, your body needs more and more oxygen. (This is why you breathe hard when you run. It is your body's natural way of getting more oxygen into your lungs.)

Some people have a tendency to hold their breath during calisthenics. *This is a very bad practice.* Not only does it defeat the value of exercise, but it can lead to dizziness or even fainting.

Breathe regularly, deeply, and at a normal pace throughout each calisthenic and each repetition.

REST BETWEEN EXERCISES    Once you have finished a series of repetitions, rest a few minutes and continue breathing deeply. A young, physically fit man may need only a few seconds to prevent any fatigue from carrying into his next exercise. An older man may need as much as three or four minutes of rest. Unfortunately, some of the "quick" physical fitness programs now on the market offer exercise methods that take just eight, ten, or twelve minutes. *This does not always make sense, because how fast one gets "winded" is highly individual.*

DON'T OVERDO REPETITIONS    Under each exercise description we give "norms" of repetitions for Programs I and II.

*No matter what program you follow, don't start out by doing the full norm of repetitions. Start with a few — perhaps three or four.* If you are not sore or tired the next day, then increase the number. (Don't be surprised if you feel a little stiff after the first time you exercise. This is natural for a man who is not in good physical condition. What we are cautioning against is not minor muscle stiffness, but deep muscle soreness or strain.)

*The secret of physical fitness lies in a slow, progressive increase of repetitions that does not place unreasonable strain on your body.*

*Note:* The suggested norms for each exercise do not apply to an older person — particularly to a man of 50 or more. He should cut the amount of repetitions in half, or do an even smaller number. At the first sign of fatigue, he should stop and rest. As necessary, he should reduce the number of repetitions to correspond to his capability.

COUNT PROPERLY    Many people lose track of the number of repetitions they have performed. All calisthenics, done on a count, should be counted as follows (our example is a 6-count exercise):

$$1 - 2 - 3 - 4 - 5 - 1$$
$$1 - 2 - 3 - 4 - 5 - 2$$
$$1 - 2 - 3 - 4 - 5 - 3$$
$$1 - 2 - 3 - 4 - 5 - 4$$
etc.

In other words, use the number of the repetition as the last count. This method will prevent your losing count in the middle of a series.

FEEL FREE TO MAKE CHANGES IN RECOMMENDED EXERCISE GROUPS    Listed below (and described later in the chapter) are so many exercises that you can devise a great many variations on the BASIC and ADVANCED groups we have suggested. But there are two points you must bear in mind:

1    Any calisthenics program should include at least one exercise for each major muscle group. (Otherwise you will overdevelop some muscles and underdevelop others.)
2    If you find that the BASIC level of calisthenics is best for you, be sure that you select only BASIC exercises — at least as a starter.

For your convenience, we have arranged the exercises below by muscle groups. Within each group, exercises are listed roughly in order of increasing difficulty.

Note that (B) indicates a BASIC exercise, and (A) an ADVANCED exercise.

# Calisthenic Exercises (by Major Muscle Groups)

## Special Calisthenic Exercises

These are the intensive exercises. Note that an advanced exercise can easily be turned into an intensive exercise by adding repetitions. The special exercises below will be useful for additional work on particular groups of muscles and to develop greater wind endurance.

On the following two pages are diagrams which show all the major muscles of your body. You will find these diagrams useful — not only for planning a schedule of calisthenics, but for choosing weight-training and isometric exercises as well. Note that muscles exist in antagonistic pairs: one *flexor* and one *extensor* muscle. When you make a movement to contract (flex) your biceps, for example, you automatically stretch (extend) your triceps muscle. It is the smooth action between muscles and nerves in per-

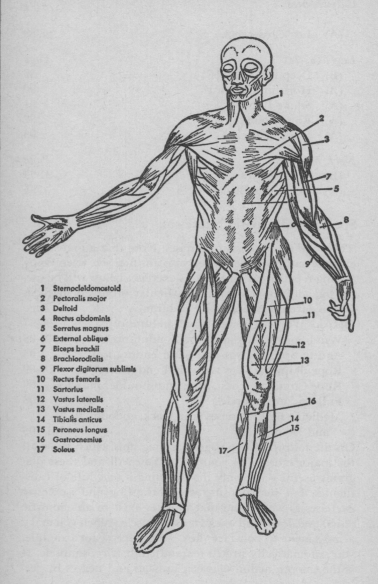

1   Sternocleidomastoid
2   Pectoralis major
3   Deltoid
4   Rectus abdominis
5   Serratus magnus
6   External oblique
7   Biceps brachii
8   Brachiorodialis
9   Flexor digitorum sublimis
10  Rectus femoris
11  Sartorius
12  Vastus lateralis
13  Vastus medialis
14  Tibialis anticus
15  Peroneus longus
16  Gastrocnemius
17  Soleus

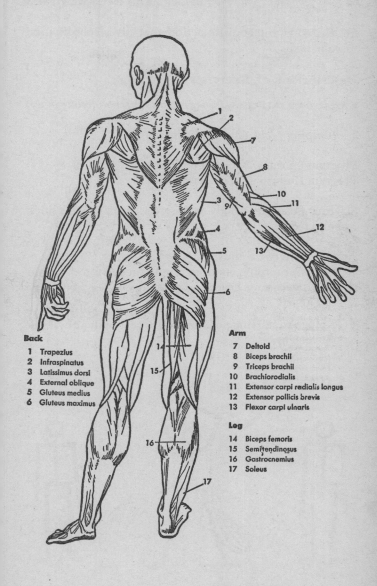

**Back**

1 Trapezius
2 Infraspinatus
3 Latissimus dorsi
4 External oblique
5 Gluteus medius
6 Gluteus maximus

**Arm**

7 Deltold
8 Biceps brachii
9 Triceps brachii
10 Brachiorodialis
11 Extensor carpi redialis longus
12 Extensor pollicis brevis
13 Flexor carpi ulnaris

**Leg**

14 Biceps femoris
15 Semitendinosus
16 Gastrocnemius
17 Soleus

forming this antagonistic action that gives coordination to your body.

## Descriptions of Exercises

WARMING-UP EXERCISES *(Benefit to all muscles of your body)*

1  *Jumping Jacks*  (Basic calisthenic)

Program I norm — 5 to 10 repetitions
Program II norm — 15 to 20 repetitions

Starting Position:   Body fully erect; arms to the sides; legs and feet together.

Action:    On two counts:
1  With a jumping motion, simultaneously touch your hands over your head, and extend your legs about two feet apart;

2  Return to starting position and repeat with a rhythmic movement.

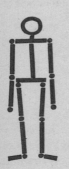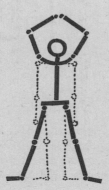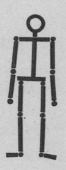

## 2 *Shadow Boxing* (Basic calisthenic)

Program I norm — 1 full minute or less
Program II norm — 2 full minutes or more

Starting Position: Body in a slight crouch; arms raised and fists clenched as in a boxer's stance; feet about shoulder-width apart and one foot a few inches forward from the other.

Action: This exercise is not done to a count. It is continuous. Starting slowly, almost in slow motion, and then increasing in tempo, throw jabs, hooks, crosses, and uppercuts. Work your feet, moving forward, backward, and to the side as a boxer does.

## 3 *Running in Place* (Advanced calisthenic)

Program I norm — 30 seconds
Program II norm — 1 full minute or longer

Starting Position: Stand erect, feet a few inches apart, weight on the balls of the feet; forearms raised in running position and parallel to the floor.

Action: Simply run in place, lifting the legs high and pumping the arms. You should start slowly, build up the pace of the exercises gradually, and then taper off speed toward the end.

## 4 *Bicycle Kick* (Advanced calisthenic)

Program I norm — 30 seconds
Program II norm — 1 full minute or longer

Starting Position: Lie on your back on a mat, a rug, or a bed; using your hands, raise your body from the hips so that your legs are up in the air and your weight rests on your shoulders and hands; brace your elbows on the mat.

**Action:** Simply simulate bicycle pedaling, moving the legs up and down. You should start slowly, build up the pace of the exercise gradually, and then taper off near the end.

This can be performed as a 2-count exercise.

1 Simultaneously raise your left leg and lower your right leg as in bicycling;

2 Reverse the action to complete the pedaling cycle — *i.e.,* raise your right leg and lower the left. Repeat with a continuous, rhythmic motion.

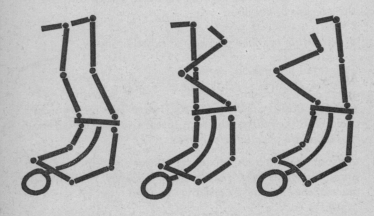

5 *Bar Hangs* (Advanced calisthenic)

Program I norm — Not recommended
Program II norm — 5 to 8 repetitions (see comments below)

**Starting Position:** Begin this exercise by hanging from a horizontal bar; be sure your feet clear the floor; your hands should be about shoulder-width apart on the bar and your feet together.

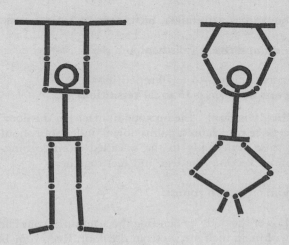

**Action:** Keeping your feet together and your knees apart, slowly pull your knees up as far as possible, similar to the motion used in the frog kick swimming stroke. Then return to the starting position, drop from the bar, rest a few seconds and repeat.

**Comments:** It is extremely important that you do not allow your body to swing. The momentum that results will interfere with the full benefits of the exercise.

This is an excellent warm-up exercise, particularly if you are then going to engage in weight training or isometrics. It is also excellent for strengthing your abdominal muscles.

*Note: These are not the only exercises you can use for warming up. Any toe touch, squatting, or stretching exercise will do a good job on your whole body, providing you perform repetitions slowly at first, then increase the pace of the exercise and taper off near the end.*

EXERCISES FOR THE CHEST, ARMS, AND SHOULDER MUSCLES

## 1  *Pushups* (Basic calisthenic)

Program I norm — 5 to 10 repetitions
Program II norm — 15 to 20 repetitions

Starting Position:   Lie on your stomach on the floor or a mat; place your hands, palms down, under your shoulders and raise your body to the so-called front leaning rest position, keeping the legs and feet together.

Action:   On two counts:

1  Lower the body by bending the arms until your chest is within an inch or two from the floor. Keep your body-line straight during the motion;

2  Return to the starting position, keeping the back straight, and repeat.

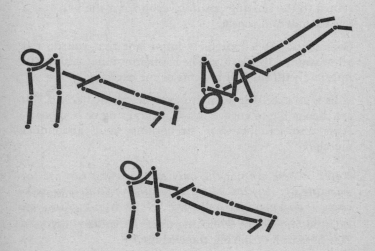

## 2 *Reverse Body Arches* (Basic calisthenic)

Program I norm — 5 to 10 repetitions
Program II norm — 15 to 20 repetitions

Starting Position: Sit on the floor, with your hands at shoulder-width and slightly behind your buttocks; keep your legs straight and together.

Action: On two counts:

1 Raise your body, arching it as high as you can, supporting your weight on your hands and heels;

2 Return to starting position and repeat.

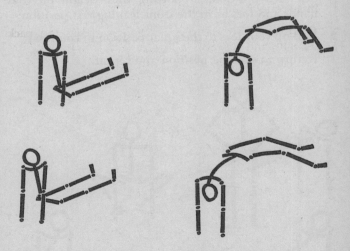

Comments: This exercise will primarily benefit your chest and upper back muscles. It also benefits your abdominal muscles by stretching them. Be sure to keep your legs out straight during the exercise.

**3**  *Squat Thrusts* (Advanced calisthenic)

Program I norm — 5 to 10 repetitions
Program II norm — 15 to 20 repetitions

Starting Position:    Body erect; hands on the hips; feet a
few inches apart.

Action:    On four counts:

1   Drop down to a squat position, hands flat on the floor,
    about shoulder-width apart and slightly in front of
    the feet;

2   Throw back your legs, keeping them together, to a fully
    extended position, supporting your weight on your
    hands and toes as in the front leaning rest position;

3   Pull up your legs to the squat position in count #1;

4   Return to starting position and repeat.

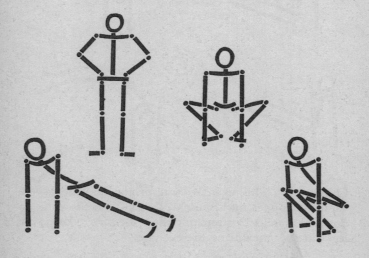

4  *Leg Kicks — from back leaning rest position*
   (Advanced calisthenic)

Program I norm — 5 to 10 repetitions
Program II norm — 15 to 20 repetitions

Starting Position:  Back leaning rest position — *i.e.,* sit on the floor, place hands about shoulder-width apart on the floor and slightly behind the buttocks; keeping the legs out straight and together, raise the body so that your back is straight, and your weight is supported on your hands and heels.

Action:  On four counts:

1  Kick left leg as high as you can into the air;

2  Return to starting position;

3  Kick right leg as high as you can into the air;

4  Return to starting position and repeat.

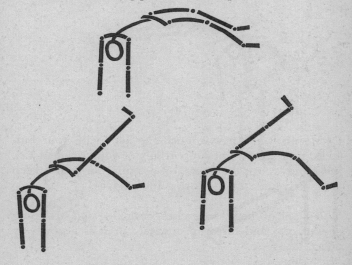

5 *Reverse Pushups* (Advanced calisthenic)

Program I norm — not recommended for this program
Program II norm — 10 to 15 repetitions

Starting Position:   Assume the back leaning rest position
described in the previous exercise.

Action:   On two counts:

1 Lower the body by bending your arms until the buttocks just touch the floor;

2 Return to starting position and repeat.

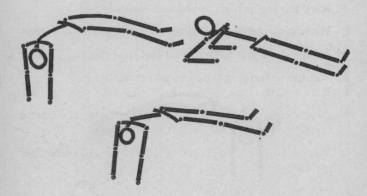

Comments:   When you touch the floor with your buttocks, they should not support any of your weight — *i.e.,*
just barely touch the floor. It is essential for you to keep
your body-line straight during this exercise.

This is one of the best exercises for flexing and stretching
your triceps and forearm muscles, but it is also a very
difficult exercise.

EXERCISES FOR THE LATERAL TRUNK MUSCLES

1  *Side Stretchers* (Basic calisthenic)

Program I norm — 5 to 10 repetitions
Program II norm — 15 to 20 repetitions

Starting Position:   Body erect; legs about shoulder-width apart; arms extended fully over the head; thumbs locked.

Action:   On eight counts:

1  Using your arms as a force, swing your body laterally to the right side, stretching the side muscles on your left;

2  With a bouncing movement, repeat the Side Stretcher on the same side;

3  Repeat once more;

4  Return to starting position;

5  Swing your body to the left side, stretching the lateral trunk muscles on your right;

6  With a bouncing movement, repeat the Side Stretcher on the same side;

7  Repeat once more;

8  Return to starting position and repeat.

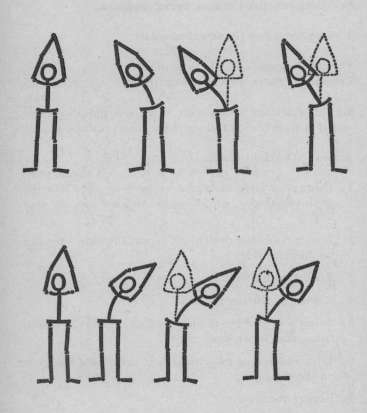

Comments:    For a slightly milder version of this exercise, omit counts 3 and 7, so that the exercise becomes a 6-count exercise. For an even milder version, omit counts 2, 3, 6, and 7, so that it becomes a 4-count exercise.

2 *Side Twisters* (Advanced calisthenic)

Program I norm — 5 to 10 repetitions
Program II norm — 15 to 20 repetitions

Starting Position: Body erect; legs slightly bent and about shoulder-width apart; arms fully extended overhead, thumbs locked.

Action: On four counts:

1 Sweep your arms down and touch the floor behind your legs;

2 With a bouncing movement, touch a point several inches outside your right foot;

3 With another bouncing movement, touch a point several inches outside your left foot;

4 Return to starting position and repeat.

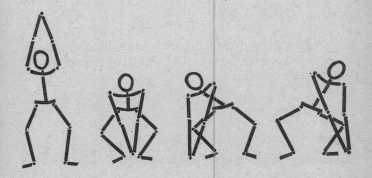

Comments:   To get the full benefits of this exercise, your body must twist when you touch outside your feet. The farther outside each foot you touch, the more stretching you give your lateral trunk muscles.

The less you bend your knees in this exercise, the more benefits your leg and back muscles also receive.

3  *Side Benders* (Advanced calisthenic)

Program I norm — 4 to 8 repetitions
Program II norm — 10 to 15 repetitions

Starting Position:   Body erect; legs straight and shoulder-width apart; arms fully extended horizontally to the sides.

Action:   On six counts:

1  Keeping arms extended horizontally, twist the trunk as far as possible to the right, using the momentum of your arms as a force;

2  With a bouncing movement, twist the body again to the right;

3  Return to starting position;

4  Twist as far as possible to the left;

5  Twist again as in count #2;

6  Return to starting position and repeat.

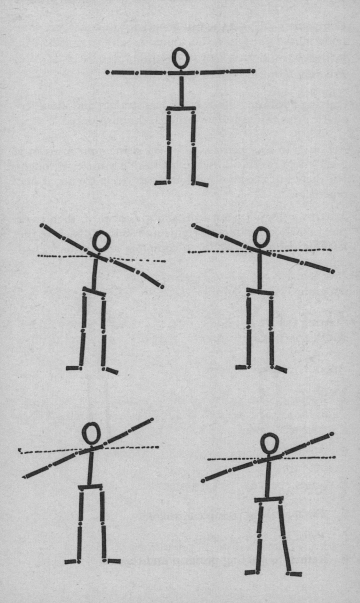

## 4  *Circle Twisters* (Advanced calisthenic)

Program I norm — 5 to 10 repetitions
Program II norm — 15 to 20 repetitions

**Starting Position:**   Body erect; legs straight and shoulder-apart; arms raised fully overhead, thumbs locked.

**Action:**   In this exercise, you will swing your arms in a great circle overhead, twisting the side muscles throughout their full range of motion. Each circle counts as one repetition.

Start by swinging your arms slightly forward, then twist them slowly around to the right, around to the back, to the left, and to the front for a complete revolution. Then repeat.

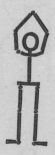    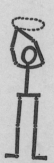

EXERCISES FOR THE BACK MUSCLES

## 1  *Toe Touchers* (Basic calisthenic)

Program I norm — 5 to 10 repetitions
Program II norm — 15 to 20 repetitions

**Starting Position:** Body erect, feet together, hands on hips.

**Action:** On two counts:

1 Bend forward from the hips and touch your toes with your fingertips. Do not bend the knees if you can possibly help it;

2 Return to starting position and repeat.

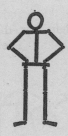 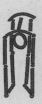 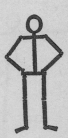

**Comments:** This exercise also gives excellent stretching to the muscles at the backs of your legs. It is primarily, however, to stretch your back muscles.

If you cannot touch your toes at first — DO NOT FORCE YOURSELF. You can either bend the knees slightly, or be content with going down only as far as you can, while keeping the knees straight. We recommend the latter course. If you keep with it, you will soon be able to touch your toes.

**2**  *Alternate Toe Touchers* (Basic calisthenic)

Program I norm — 5 to 10 repetitions
Program II norm — 15 to 20 repetitions

Starting Position:    Body erect, legs about shoulder-width apart; arms fully extended horizontally to the sides.

Action:    On four counts:

1   Bending the body forward from the hips, cross over the right hand and touch the left toe;

2   Return to starting position;

3   Cross over the left hand and touch the right toe;

4   Return to starting position and repeat.

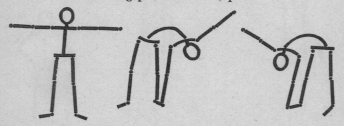

Comments:    To receive the full benefit of this exercise, you should keep your legs straight.

Note that the Alternate Toe Toucher does not give you quite as much back stretching as the regular Toe Toucher. In the Alternate Toe Toucher, your legs are spread slightly apart, in effect moving you "closer to your toes."

**3**  *Back Stretchers* (Advanced calisthenic)

Program I norm — 4 to 8 repetitions
Program II norm — 15 to 20 repetitions

Starting Position:   Body erect; legs straight but spread about shoulder-width apart; arms fully extended overhead; thumbs locked.

Action:   On four counts:

1   Sweep the arms down and touch the floor between your feet, bending your knees slightly;

2   With a bouncing movement, touch the floor behind your feet, as far back as possible;

3   Bounce again and touch the floor behind your feet — again, as far back as possible;

4   Return to starting position and repeat.

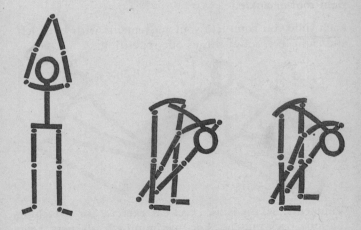

Remember that **YOU MUST NEVER FORCE MUSCLES BEYOND THEIR ABILITIES**. If you cannot do this exercise at first with your legs straight, do not make the mistake of lunging down, putting an extreme strain on your muscles. This could result in torn or injured muscles.

4   *Sitting Back Stretchers* (Advanced calisthenic)

Program I norm — 3 to 6 repetitions
Program II norm — 10 to 15 repetitions

Starting Position:   Sit on the floor, legs apart at about a 45-degree angle; hands on the hips.

Action:   This is not an exercise that works best with a rhythmic count.

Reach forward and grasp your left ankle or foot (depending on how far you can reach), bending the trunk as close to the left thigh as possible. Rock forward several times, grasping the foot or ankle each time. Then repeat with the right foot or ankle.

Each time you complete your movements with both left and right feet, count this as one repetition.

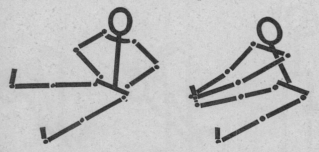

Comments:   This is an excellent exercise for stretching the long back muscles. For maximum effectiveness, keep the legs straight throughout the exercise.

A variation on this exercise is to reach forward and simultaneously grasp the left foot or ankle with the left hand, the right foot or ankle with the right hand, and try to touch your forehead to the floor between your legs.

EXERCISES FOR THE ABDOMINAL MUSCLES

1  *Leg-ups* (Basic calisthenic)

Program I norm — 5 to 10 repetitions
Program II norm — 15 to 20 repetitions

Starting Position:   Lie on your back; arms at sides; legs straight, and feet together.

Action:   On two counts:

1  Raise feet together to a point perpendicular to the floor;

2  Return to starting position and repeat.

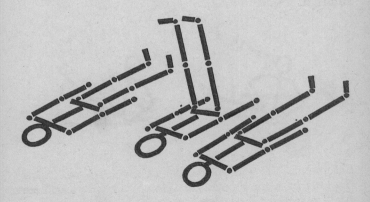

Comments:   Your abdominal muscles should do the work here, not your arms or elbows.

**2**  *Scissors* (Basic calisthenic)

**Program I norm** — 5 to 10 repetitions
**Program II norm** — 15 to 20 repetitions

**Starting Position:**  Sit on the floor with upper body erect or leaning slightly back for balance; legs should be fully extended, slightly apart and lifted two to three inches off the floor; hands on hips.

**Action:**  On two counts:

1  Raise left leg about six inches, while simultaneously lowering right leg;

2  Reverse the action — *i.e.*, raise right leg about six inches above the starting position, while simultaneously lowering the left, then repeat.

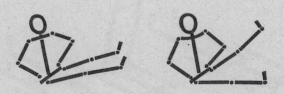

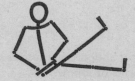

Comments: This is a continuous exercise — *i.e.,* do not return to the starting position at the end of each repetition. To get added benefits, increase the pace of this exercise as you progress in your training.

You can turn this exercise into a very vigorous one by quickening the pace to a point that is comparable to that of a rapid stationary run.

3 *Sit-ups* (Advanced calisthenic)

Program I norm — 4 to 8 repetitions
Program II norm — 10 to 20 repetitions

Starting Position: Lie flat on the floor, legs together; arms clasped behind the head; anchor your feet.

Action: On two counts:

1 Raise your upper body from the hips to a sitting position, using the power of your abdominal muscles; touch your left elbow to your right knee;

2 Return to starting position and repeat.

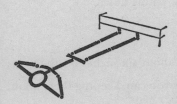 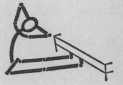

Comments: This is one of the few exercises that can get confusing. On the first repetition, touch your left elbow to your right knee; on the following repetition touch your right elbow to the left knee. Then alternate knees on successive repetitions.

For full effect, your feet must be anchored — under a radiator, a sofa, or whatever stationary object is handy. If you practice with a partner, he can hold your feet.

4  *Leg Splits* (Advanced calisthenic)

Program I norm — not recommended
Program II norm — 6 to 12 repetitions

Starting Position: Lie flat on your back, feet and legs together; arms at your sides, palms down.

Action:  On four counts:

1  Raise both legs together about six inches off the floor;

2  Spread legs apart as far as you can, keeping them about six inches off the floor;

3  Return to position as in count #1;

4  Return to starting position and repeat.

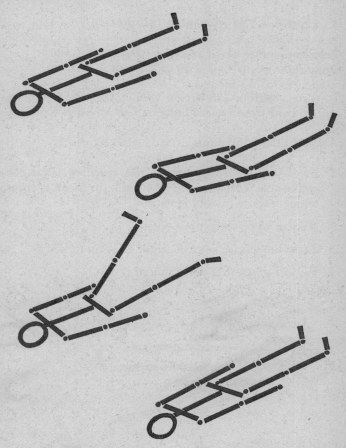

**Comments:** For full effect, you must exercise at a slow pace — about two seconds for each count or longer. Interestingly enough, raising the legs about six inches off the floor and holding them for about five seconds is roughly approximate to a weight-training, and, in a sense, to an isometric exercise. The weight of your legs puts force or weight on your abdominal muscles.

5  *Leg Crossovers* (Advanced calisthenic)

Program I norm — not recommended
Program II norm — 10 to 15 repetitions

Starting Position: Lie flat on your back; arms extended straight out from your shoulders; feet and legs together.

Action:   On four counts:

1  Cross your right leg over the left, reaching as far out as possible with your leg and trying to touch a point about level with your waist;

2  Return to starting position;

3  Cross the left leg over the right as in count #1;

4  Return to starting position and repeat.

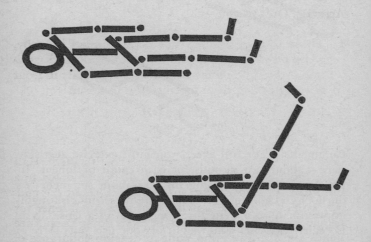

Comments: Keep your shoulders flat on the floor throughout this exercise. Also, try to keep the stationary leg as straight as possible while you cross the other one over it.

A variation is to start with both legs together, straight up in the air, then cross first to one side and then the other.

EXERCISES FOR THE LEG MUSCLES

1 *Deep Knee Bends* (Basic calisthenic)

Program I norm — 5 to 10 repetitions
Program II norm — 15 to 20 repetitions

Starting Position: Body erect; hands on hips; heels together, toes pointing outward at approximately a 45-degree angle.

Action: On two counts:

1 Throw your weight onto the balls of your feet (actually, go up on your toes) as you drop into a full squat position. At the same time, extend your arms fully in front of you, keeping them together, palms down;

2 Return to starting position and repeat.

Comments: A variation of this exercise is called "Half Knee Bends." In this exercise, you do not go down to a full squat position; rather, you go only to about the midway point. This variation is useful as a conditioner for people who have trouble when they start doing Deep Knee Bends and for those who want to develop endurance of extensor muscles of their upper legs.

2   *Horizontal Sprint* (Basic calisthenic)

Program I norm — 5 to 10 repetitions
Program II norm — 15 to 20 repetitions

Starting Position:   Assume a full squat position; then
extend the left leg fully to the rear; arms should be
straight, fingers pointing to the front; head held high.

Action:   On two counts:

1   Simultaneously bring the left leg forward as far as you
    can, and extend the right leg fully back;

2   Reverse the action in count #1 so that you return to
    the starting position; then repeat.

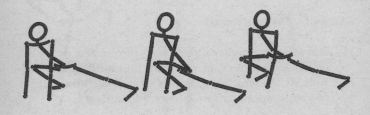

Comments:   As a muscle-conditioning calisthenic, this
exercise can be done at any pace. This is also an excellent
warm-up exercise for Program II or Program III. In this
case, you should start slowly and gradually build up the
pace to the point where you are virtually sprinting in
place — then taper off. A good exercise level is one to two
minutes of continuous Horizontal Sprints.

**3**  *Squat Jumps* (Advanced calisthenic)

Program I norm — 5 to 10 repetitions
Program II norm — 15 to 20 repetitions

Starting Position:  Assume a full squat position; legs about six inches apart, and the left foot slightly in front of the right; weight should be on the balls of your feet; clasp your hands over your head.

Action:   On two counts:

1  Spring into the air as far as possible, reversing the order of your feet and straightening the legs;

2  Return to starting position, but with the right foot slightly in front of the left; then repeat.

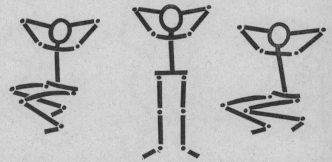

Comments:   In this exercise you reverse the order of your feet in successive repetitions in much the same manner as you reverse elbow touches in Sit-ups.

For full effect, you must jump as high as you can each time. The great benefit of this exercise is that it causes a good deal of both stretching and flexing of your leg muscles.

We recommend that anyone use this exercise in Program I only with caution, for it is uncommonly strenuous.

4  *Kangaroo Hops* (Advanced calisthenic)

Program I norm — 5 to 10 repetitions
Program II norm — 15 to 20 repetitions

Starting Position:  Body in half crouch with legs bent and back straight; hands on the hips; feet slightly apart and weight on balls of feet.

Action:  On two counts:

1  Jump up and forward as far as you can;
2  Return to half-squatting position as you land; then repeat.

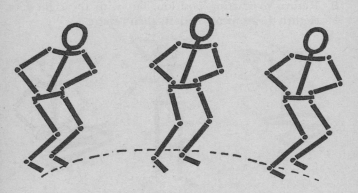

Comments:  As you jump, keep your legs bent and your back straight. Otherwise you could lose your balance and fall on your face. Resist the temptation to sink into a low squat on landing. For full effect, you must keep your legs bent in an approximately half squat or crouched position throughout repetitions.

Because of its sudden motions, we recommend the use of this exercise in Program I only with caution.

## 5  *Russian Kicks* (Advanced calisthenic)

Program I norm — not recommended
Program II norm — 10 to 15 repetitions

Starting Position:   Full squat; feet about six inches apart and weight on the balls of the feet; hands on hips.

Action:   On four counts:

1  Kick left leg out to full extension, just touching heel to floor;

2  Return to starting position;

3  Kick right leg out;

4  Return to starting position and repeat.

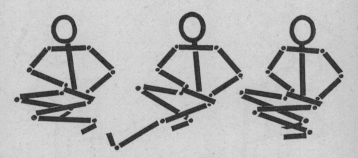

Comments:   This exercise not only benefits all the muscles in your legs, but is also excellent for developing balance.

A variation of this exercise is to perform it in a continuous motion, but this is extremely strenuous. It may look easy when you see a Russian dancer do it, but try it once and you will see that it is one of the most difficult exercises in this book.

**EXERCISES FOR THE NECK MUSCLES**

1   *Neck Flex* (Basic calisthenic)

Program I norm — 3 to 6 repetitions, each position
Program II norm — 8 to 12 repetitions, each position

Starting Position:   Body erect, feet together, arms at sides.

Action:   On four counts, bend the neck forward and try to touch the chin to the chest. With a bouncing motion, repeat two more times and return to the starting position;

Then repeat to the right and left and backward.

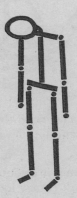
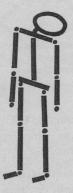

Comments:   This is an excellent exercise for improving posture, since the neck muscles play a vital role in maintaining good posture.

2   *Wrestler's Bridge* (Advanced calisthenic)

Program I norm — not recommended
Program II norm — 10 to 15 repetitions

Starting Position:   Lie flat on the floor; feet together with knees drawn up comfortably so soles rest flat on the floor; extend arms to the sides, straight out from the shoulders.

Action:   On two counts:

1   Raise and arch your body as far as you can, supporting your weight on your head and soles of the feet;

2   Return to the starting position and repeat.

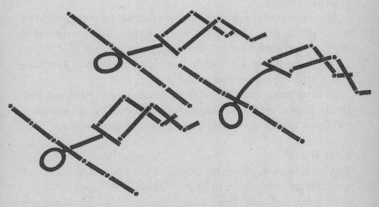

Comments:   It is important that you do not use your arms and hands to raise your weight. Your arms should be used for balance only.

SPECIAL EXERCISES (MISCELLANEOUS)

We include these exercises particularly for people interested in Program III — *i.e.,* those who want more work on building up endurance of particular muscles, those who want to improve their wind endurance, and those who simply want more strenuous exercises. Because there are so few of these exercises, we do not classify them by groups of muscles. Rather, under each exercise, we simply describe its purpose and benefits.

*Roadwork* (To increase endurance of your leg muscles and your wind)

Here is a fairly intensive roadwork program based on one used by the Dallas Cowboys. This is a fine program, if you are already in good condition; it will do wonders for your wind within six weeks. People who are not in good condition, however, should adopt a much more moderate and gradual program.

Note that this program aims at intensive development of wind endurance over a six-week period. Remember that NFL players who follow this program, or one like it, are going to be doing a great deal of running during training camp and the regular season.

If you decide to follow this program you should not suddenly stop after six weeks, but continue with the schedule outlined under the sixth week as a regular routine.

*First Week**
Jog a mile or more each day; include some hill-climbing on your route, or add some stair-running to your schedule.

*Second Week**
Two 440s† — sprint
Two 880s — jog
Four 220s—three-quarter speed

* Based on a five-day week.
† All distances are expressed in yards.

*Third Week\**
Two 440s — sprint
One 880 — jog
One mile — one-half speed

*Fourth Week\**
Run a mile each day, striving for 90-second quarters.

*Fifth Week\**
Two 440s — sprint
One 880 — jog
Five 220s — three-quarter speed
Six 40s — sprint

*Sixth Week\**
Two 440s — sprint
Six 220s — three-quarter speed
Ten 40s — sprint

Comments:  Never perform roadwork exercise without first warming up, particularly if a series starts out with a sprint. (Jogging is a perfectly good warm-up.)

*Wind Sprints* (To increase endurance of your leg muscles and your wind)

These may be done in a variety of ways to develop your wind and leg endurance, and to keep them in condition. Here are two possibilities:

1  (In a limited area, at least a hundred yards long.)
a  Jog the full distance and back;
b  Run the full distance at half-speed and jog back;
c  Run the full distance at a sprint and jog back;
d  Sprint half the distance and jog the remainder at least five round trips.

2  (On the road.)
a  Jog first for at least a quarter of a mile. Then run 50 yards at half speed and jog 100 yards. Do this twice;
b  Then run a series of 50-yard sprints followed by a 100-yard jog for as many repetitions as you can do without approaching exhaustion.

One advantage of this technique (which also may be applied to Wind Sprints in an enclosed area) is that you have a built-in measure of your progress keeping track of repetitions.

*Agility Sprints* (To improve coordination)

These are particularly good for athletes who must make many sudden changes in direction — right, left, forward, back-pedaling, etc. — during a game.

1 Start by jogging at least 200 yards; then run 50 yards at half speed and jog 50 more yards; then run at least three repetitions of 50-yard sprints followed by 50-yard jogs;

2 *Back pedal:* Back pedal at full speed, break at right angles and keep back pedaling — 10 yards for each direction. Run this exercise for at least 100 yards;

3 *Cuts:* Run straight ahead at about half speed for about 25 yards. Practice cutting two ways: one by cutting left, pushing off on your right foot; another by crossing one leg over the other to change direction;

4 *Half turns:* Run 10 yards at full speed, jump in the air, do a half turn, then back pedal at full speed. Repeat at least 10 times.

*Rope Skipping* (Primarily builds leg muscle endurance)

This exercise is not strenuous in itself. Its value comes from the length of time you exercise. A well-conditioned athlete can rope skip almost indefinitely at about a jog pace. Be sure to get a rope that is long enough but not too long to drag over the floor on the down stroke. Ideally, the rope should just touch the floor as you swing it naturally.

Rope Skipping can be done two ways:

1 Both feet come off the floor at once. (This gives more exercise to your upper leg muscles, particularly the extensors.)

2   Feet alternate, in rhythm. (This gives more exercise to your lower leg muscles, or calves.)

You may find a little practice is required to perfect your coordination in this exercise.

*Rope Climbing* (Develops arm, shoulder, back, and abdominal muscles)

This is a wonderful exercise for building your upper body. It is really a combination of a calisthenic and a weight-training exercise because your body itself acts as weight.

But proceed with caution. More than a few people have misjudged their ability the first time around and have lost their grip 15 to 20 feet off the floor — sustaining painful rope burns or a bad fall — so practice this exercise slowly. Start with a climb to about ten feet, then increase the height gradually until you build up to the full height. The height of the rope can vary from 15 to 40 feet. The usual height is about 25 feet.

Be sure that the climbing rope is well anchored overhead. This is no place for do-it-yourself unless you have skilled supervision. The best place to do Rope Climbing is in a gymnasium or a health club where professional climbing anchors are used.

All action should be in the shoulders and arms. Your feet should be together and should not flail about during the climb.

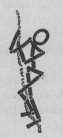 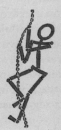 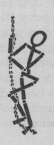

*Pull-ups* (Benefit arm, shoulder, chest, and abdominal
   muscles)

We include this exercise under special exercises because,
like several of the other special exercises, it is really a
cross between a calisthenic and a weight-training exercise.
The weight of the body acts as resistance.

You will need a stout bar which is high enough so your
feet do not touch the floor when you are at full hang. If
you make your own, be sure the bar is strong enough (a
stout pipe, or preferably a solid steel bar, well mounted).
Be careful about this: Some people blithely assume that because a bar *looks* strong, it *is* strong. Horizontal bars will of
course be available in most health clubs and gymnasiums.

To perform the exercise, start from the full hang, with
hands about shoulder-width apart, palms away from the
body.

The action of the exercise is to raise the body with the
arms and shoulders until the chin is even with the bar.
You should not put your chin over the bar and rest any of
your weight on it. This would defeat the purpose of the
exercise. Do not let your body swing. You should go
straight up and come straight down. Your legs should not
flail about or swing out in front.

Performing the exercise on two counts, aim to build up
repetitions over a period of time. Ten full Pull-ups is a satisfactory number of repetitions. This is a difficult exercise
for most people. Exercising in "sets" is a good way of increasing the benefits you receive from Pull-ups. Suppose
you can perform only eight Pull-ups with relative ease;
try performing three sets of five Pull-ups each, resting a
couple of minutes between sets.

A variation of this exercise is to place your hands on the
bar with the palms toward you. This does not give as
much general exercise to your entire arm muscles, but it
does put an emphasis on your biceps muscles.

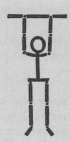 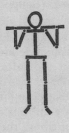

**MEDICINE BALL EXERCISES** (Various muscles as indicated)

All medicine ball exercises are designed for use with a partner, since it is pretty difficult to get much good out of the medicine ball working alone.

1  *Arm Push* (Benefits abdominal, chest, and arm muscles)

Starting Position:   One man sits and holds the medicine ball overhead; feet about ten inches apart; the other man stands between his legs and places his hands on the top of the medicine ball.

Action:   Move the ball up and down in rhythmic motion with your hands while your partner pushes down for 20 to 40 repetitions; then change places and repeat the exercise.

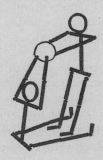

2  *Leg Push* (Benefits abdominal and leg muscles)

Starting Position:   Lie on your back; pull up your legs as in a semi-bicycle kick position; have your partner place the ball on the soles of your feet.

Action:   Exercising in rhythm, move the ball up and down with your legs as your partner pushes down for 20 to 40 repetitions; then reverse positions and repeat the exercise.

3  *Overhead Throw* from sitting position (Benefits chest, abdominal, and arm muscles)

Starting Position:   Partners sit on the floor, facing each other about 15 feet apart; legs should be about 18 inches apart.

Action:   Partners toss ball back and forth with an overhead motion, catching the ball overhead the same way, for about 20 to 40 repetitions.

4  *Leaning Throw* (Benefits back, leg, abdominal, and arm muscles)

Starting Position:   Partners stand about 20 feet apart. Each leans forward from the waist; feet about two feet apart; body in a semi-crouch.

Action:   The partners toss the ball back and forth. The point of the exercise is to catch the ball, swing it back between your legs and throw it forward again — all in one continuous motion, keeping the ball about two feet off the floor during the whole exercise. Again, perform about 20 to 40 repetitions.

5   *Chest Snaps* (Benefits pectoral and arm muscles)

Starting Position:   Two people stand about 15 to 20 feet apart.

Action:   Snap the ball back and forth from chest height, as in throwing a basketball. Perform about 20 to 40 repetitions. This exercise is also very good for the wrist muscles.

Further calisthenic exercises of a special nature may be found in this book. See the chapter POSTURE, for special corrective exercises; the chapter WEIGHT CONTROL, for exercises which will help you gain or lose weight; the chapter SPORTS, for exercises which help you develop the muscles used in certain sports.

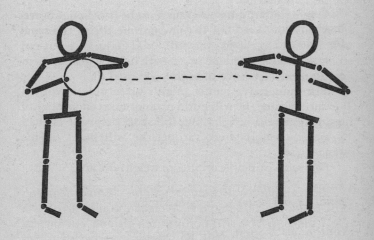

# 7

## WEIGHT TRAINING

The purpose of weight training is to increase your strength scientifically, by pitting your muscles against progressively greater resistance.

George Menefee, trainer of the Los Angeles Rams, offers a simple explanation:

"A strength-building program must be based on progressively increased weights. If you continue lifting the same weight week after week, you will build endurance but not strength. Muscles increase in strength only by pitting them against more resistance than they are used to.

"If a man plays tennis month after month with a 14-ounce racquet, he will build up enormous endurance of his arm and wrist muscles. But if he goes progressively to a 15- and then a 16-ounce racquet, he will build up his strength, too.

"This same principle applies to weight training."

Weight training requires *equipment* (*see* "Equipment You Will Need," in this chapter). Weight training involves a new idea: *sets*. You still perform repetitions, but in sets, — or *groups of repetitions*. For instance; rather than perform 20 repetitions of an exercise, you perform two sets of 10 repetitions each, with a short rest between sets. This prevents overtaxing your muscles. We offer three groups of weight-training exercises — BASIC, ADVANCED, and INTENSIVE — just as we did with calisthenics.

## The BASIC Group

Included are a weight-training warm-up and eight exercises which will give strength-building, body-building, and endurance-building benefits to all the muscles of your body.

Before you begin:

*Repetitions:* We recommend *two sets of 5 repetitions* for each exercise, to be gradually increased to *two sets of 8 repetitions.*

*Choosing your weights:* How much weight you should lift depends upon your age, strength, and endurance — as well as the difficulty of each exercise.

However, we offer a general guide for those following the BASIC group of exercises:

Start with 25 to 50 pounds for exercises which involve

your upper body muscles (Arm Curls, Presses, etc.), and 40 to 80 pounds for exercises which primarily involve your leg muscles (Squats, Rise-on-toes, etc.).

This general guide will apply to eight out of every ten men. However, if even the lowest suggested weight seems too heavy, then lessen the amount, until you can *comfortably* perform two sets of 5 repetitions. Your muscles should feel "used up," but not strained or exhausted. If on the other hand these weights are too light, then experiment by *gradually* adding weight, until you find the poundage which enables you *comfortably* to perform your two sets of 5 repetitions.

*Increasing Repetitions and Weight:* As you develop strength, first increase your repetitions gradually from 5 to 8. Then progressively add weight in small amounts — five pounds at a time for upper body·muscles, 10 pounds for leg muscles.

## The ADVANCED Group

This group includes a weight-training warm-up and nine exercises. Some of these exercises are more difficult than those in the BASIC group. But the primary difference lies in *increased repetitions and heavier weights*.

Before you begin:

(5) Pullover (chest)                                 125-26
(6) Sit-ups (abdominal)                           129-30
(7) Rise-on-toes (calves)                        134-35
(8) Front or Shoulder Squat (thighs and hips)    130-32
(9) Rowing (upper back and arms)               118

*Repetitions:* We recommend two sets of 7 repetitions — to be gradually increased to *two sets of 10 repetitions.*

*Choosing Your Weights:* This will not be a problem, since you will have progressed from a BASIC group of exercises. Simply use the same poundage to which you progressed in your BASIC exercises.

*Increasing Repetitions and Weights:* Follow the same two principles of progression suggested for the BASIC group:

First, advance gradually from 7 to 10 repetitions. Then increase weight 5 pounds at a time for upper body muscles, and 10 pounds for leg muscles.

When faced with new or radically different exercies, you must rely upon intelligent experimentation. (The Dead Lift, involving heavier poundage than any BASIC exercise, is a good example.)

Using the "safety-first" approach, begin experimenting with a very light weight. Then *gradually* add weight until you find the poundage which allows you to *comfortably* perform two sets of 7 repetitions.

## The INTENSIVE Group

Included are a weight-training warm-up and ten exercises. Some of the exercises are more difficult than those in the ADVANCED group, but the primary differences are *more sets and heavier weights.*

Before you begin:

                                     *Page*
(a) Calisthenics (at least 5 minutes);         64-66

*Repetitions:* We recommend *three sets of 7 repetitions*
— to be gradually increased to *three sets of 10 repetitions.*

*Choosing Your Weights:* Anyone reaching the INTEN-
SIVE level of exercises will have progressed from the
ADVANCED group.

But since you will now be expending far more effort by
performing *three sets* of repetitions rather than two, you
must make an adjustment in the poundage you lift.
Decrease the weights for exercises involving the upper
body muscles by 10 to 20 pounds, and for exercises
involving the leg muscles by 20 to 30 pounds — at least as
a start.

*Increasing Repetitions and Weights:* As you become
used to performing three sets, you can gradually add the
poundage which you substracted as you started on your
INTENSIVE group of exercises.

As your strength continues to increase, simply follow
the same two principles of progression as applied to the
BASIC and ADVANCED exercise groups: First, advance
gradually from 7 to 10 repetitions. Then add weight 5
pounds at a time for upper body muscles, and 10 pounds
for leg muscles.

Fred Zamberletti, trainer of the Minnesota Vikings, explains why most people should stick to 7 to 10 repetitions as a maximum for each set:

"I believe that 7 to 10 repetitions are ideal for any man who pursues a fairly strenuous weight-training program. More repetitions would put too much emphasis on endurance; fewer repetitions would not offer enough endurance-building exercise.

"If a man does only a few repetitions — maybe 3 or 4 — he's probably going to be working with very heavy weights. This is a dangerous practice that throws too much emphasis on strength without the necessary development of endurance. Strength without endurance is an artificial concept of physical fitness."

## How To Perform Weight-Training Exercises

FOLLOW DIRECTIONS EXACTLY
Weight training often involves strenuous moves, working against considerable weight. There is no particular danger involved as long as you do the exercises correctly, and without attempting to lift too heavy a weight.

ALWAYS WARM UP   Before starting a weight-training session, you should perform at least 5 minutes of calisthenic warm-ups. Immediately before starting your exercises, you should always perform the special weight-training warm-up. This exercise, using actual weights, will work your muscles in stages and get them fully prepared for more strenuous lifting.

WARNING: DON'T TREAT ALL YOUR MUSCLES ALIKE   The principle of gradually increased weights will benefit every muscle in your body. *But you must choose weights according to the strength of your muscles.* Your leg and back muscles are the strongest in your body: the legs because they receive constant exercise just from walking and carrying your body weight; the back muscles because they, too, help support your weight in normal posture. (It is interesting to note that a very powerful man, who may be able to exert 600 pounds of force with his arms, can apply nearly 2,000 pounds with his legs.)

Your arm, stomach, shoulder, and lateral trunk muscles are much weaker than your leg and back muscles. As a result they can be developed more quickly. For relatively undeveloped muscles offer far more "room for improvement."

*A Problem: "Sticking Points"*    Normally, as you progress with a weight-training exercise, you will progressively add small weights while you continue to do the same number of repetitions.

But eventually you will reach a point where you cannot add any more weight to the barbell, without being forced to decrease your number of repetitions.

This is the "sticking point."

Do not decrease the number of repetitions. Instead, do one of two things:

1    *Try a different exercise.* It will necessarily exercise your muscles in a slightly different way.

2    *Vary your sets, using heavier weights.* For example, if you are stuck on three sets of 10 repetitions using a 150-pound weight, try

> 8 repetitions — 140 pounds
>
> 6 repetitions — 165 pounds
>
> 3 repetitions — 180 pounds

Since such possibilities are endless, you will have to experiment carefully to discover which combination is perfect for you.

NEVER BEND YOUR BACK WHEN PICKING UP A BARBELL    The correct movement for lifting a barbell from the floor is that used in the weight-training warm-up. Be sure to read the instructions for this exercise before you lift any weights.

Perhaps you've heard certain terms used in competitive weight-training — the clean and jerk, or the snatch. We suggest that you do not attempt to use such strenuous movements except under professional supervision. We are concerned only with getting the barbell to an exercise position safely, not with techniques for lifting a large mass of weight with a classical movement.

DON'T LET YOUR BODY DEVELOP MOMENTUM   You may tend to develop a "rhythm," or body swing, in certain exercises. This will prevent you from receiving the full benefits of such exercises, for your body momentum will be "lifting" a part of the weight.

The way to avoid this bad habit is always to come to a full stop between each repetition of an exercise.

REST BETWEEN SETS   No matter what your level of physical fitness, you must always rest between sets. We suggest a minimum resting perod of 3 to 5 minutes for the average man, otherwise you will go into the next exercise with your muscles in a state of partial fatigue, which will prevent you from receiving the full benefits of the exercise. (But do not rest so long that your muscles get "cold.")

BREATHE PROPERLY   There is nothing wrong with holding your breath during an exercise, for under the stress of lifting a heavy weight, normal breathing is impossible.

We suggest that you take a deep breath when you start an exercise, then hold it as you lift the weight, and exhale towards the end of the repetition.

When first you start weight training, do not hold your breath for longer than 3 to 4 seconds. And *never* hold it longer than 8 seconds, no matter how proficient you become.

DON'T EXERCISE EVERY DAY   No matter what group of exercises you follow, you should exercise only three times a week — every other day (perhaps Monday, Wednesday, and Friday).

Each "day off" from lifting is necessary to give your muscles a chance to take advantage of the body-building benefits of each exercise.

DON'T TAKE ANY RISKS   Treat even small weights with respect.

*Never* tape your hands to the bar to help you handle heavier weights.

*Never* lie under flimsy weight racks. Use only carefully tested, sturdy equipment.

THERE IS NOTHING WRONG WITH SENSIBLE IMPROVISING

If you get bored with one exercise, feel free to substitute another which benefits the same muscles. Some exercises are more difficult than others, however, so be sure to match weights to your ability.

No matter what group of exercises you follow, *you should always include calisthenics, a weight-training warm-up, and one exercise for each muscle group.*

## Weight-Training Exercises (by Major Muscle Groups)

You will note that there are more "muscle groups" for weight training than there are for calisthenics. This is because weight training gives intensive exercise to fewer muscles at one time.

## Equipment You Will Need

If you do not belong to a gym or health club, you will have to invest in equipment:

1 *A barbell:* a solid steel shaft, 4 to 6 feet long, with collars which screw on to secure weights firmly to each end;

2 *An assortment of weights* of different poundage which fit onto the barbell;

3 *A sturdy bench,* about 16 inches high and 6 feet long;

4  Mats for the bench (for comfort) and for the floor (to protect it); position the mats about 30 inches apart and stand between them, so the weights can rest on the mats;

5  *Two sturdy racks* to hold the barbell, one at waist level and one at shoulder level (because many exercises start at these heights).

6  *Optional equipment:* This includes *leg weights* (sandals which have reinforced holes to hold a short bar with weights), *neck weights* (headgear which holds weights), and *dumbbells.*

To keep the number of exercises down to a reasonable and manageable number, most of the exercises in this book require only a barbell. The few exercises we include involving optional equipment offer unusually fine benefits. (In case this equipment is unavailable to you, we have included a barbell exercise which offers approximately the same benefits.)

## Detailed Instructions for Weight-Training Exercises

The question of how much weight to lift has been fully covered earlier in the chapter. However, to insure that you receive maximum benefit from every exercise you perform, we indicate in each exercise diagram whether you should use heavier or lighter weights than "normal."

THE WEIGHT-TRAINING WARM-UP *(To work all muscles in stages)*

Weights:   Select weights well within your lifting capacity.
Starting Position:   Stand close to the barbell (your shins should actually brush it); keep your feet on a line and about a foot apart; lower your hips so that your buttocks

are low; grasp the barbell with your palms toward your legs and at shoulder-width.

Action: (A) On two counts:

1 *Keeping your back straight,* lift the barbell and straighten up fully. Your arms should then be fully extended downward ("at the hang") with the barbell resting across your thighs. Let your legs do the initial lifting when you first raise the barbell;

2 Lower the barbell to the floor, *keeping your back straight,* and repeat 3 to 5 times.

(B) On two counts, continue:

1 Starting with the barbell at the hang, pull it up fully to your chest;

2 Lower to the hang position and repeat 3 to 5 times. (Do not set the barbell down during this exercise. If you are unable to sustain the repetitions, you have selected weights that are too heavy, and you should lighten them.)

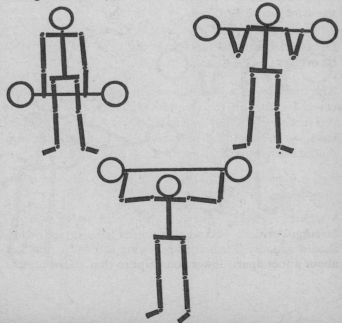

(C) On two counts, continue:

1  Without setting the barbell down, pull it up fully to your chest from the hang position and press it overhead;

2  Return the barbell to chest level and repeat 3 to 5 times.

Comments: Properly executed, this warm-up exercise will fully prepare your body for weight training by working your muscles progressively in stages.

### EXERCISES FOR THE NECK MUSCLES

*Wrestler's Bridge*

Weights: Considerably lighter than average.

Starting Position: Same as the calisthenic except that you hold the barbell above your chest. Hands about shoulder-width apart; palms away from your body.

Action: On two counts:

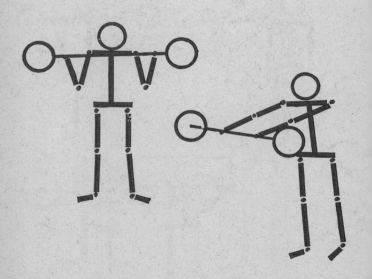

1   At the same time you assume the wrestler's bridge
    position, press the barbell to full-arm extension;
2   Return to starting position and repeat.

Comments:   This is one of the very few conventional
barbell exercises which gives primary benefits to the neck
muscles.

Another exercise (of a special type) for neck muscles is as
follows:

Using headgear to hold small weights, you can adapt the
Neck Flex calisthenic to a weight-training exercise. Be
careful to use only light weights.

### EXERCISES FOR THE UPPER BACK AND ARMS

1   *Shoulder Shrugs*

Weights:   Heavier than average.
Starting Position:   Start with the barbell at the hang
position.
Action:   On two counts:
1   Shrug your shoulders as high as possible, keeping your
    arms at the hang position; rotate your shoulders for-
    ward and backward with a circular motion.
2   Return to starting position and repeat.

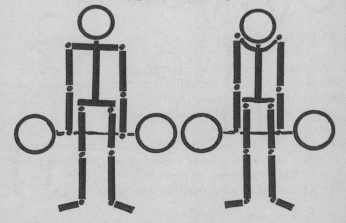

### 2  Rowing

**Weights:**  Lighter than average.
**Starting Position:**  Start with the barbell at the hang position; then lean forward from the hips so that your upper body is horizontal with the floor; allow barbell to hang with your arms fully extended (it will be a few inches off the floor); your hands should be about shoulder-width apart; palms toward your body; your feet about two feet apart.
**Action:**  On two counts:
1  With no motion of your legs or body, pull the barbell up to a point just under your pectoral muscles;
2  Return to starting position and repeat.


**Comments:**  You may find it helpful to use a chair in this exercise to be sure your upper body is in the correct horizontal position. There is nothing wrong with actually resting your head on the back of the chair at first, providing you do not let your head support your weight.


### 3  Upright Rowing

**Weights:**  Lighter than average.
**Starting Position:**  Barbell at the hang position; your hands should be close together (about twelve inches apart), with the palms toward your body.
**Action:**  On two counts:
1  Keeping your legs and body straight throughout the exercise and your elbows higher than the barbell, pull the barbell straight up to your chin;
2  Return to starting position and repeat.

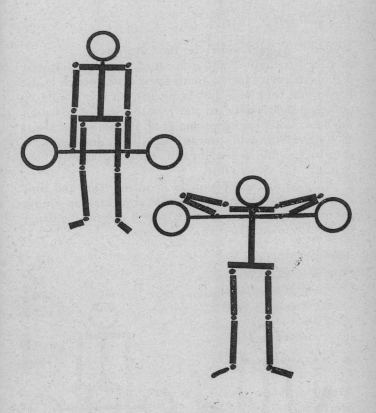

Comments:   You can put your hands closer together and receive added benefits from this exercise — the closer the better (but not closer than three inches; you will begin to lose control over the barbell if your hands get too close together). Another exercise to benefit your back and arm muscles is to attach a weight to your belt and perform pull-ups.

EXERCISES FOR THE LOWER BACK AND HIPS

## 1 *Dead Lift*

Weight:    Average to heavier than average.
Starting Position:    Stand in front of a barbell with your feet about twelve inches apart; stand close enough to the bar so that your shins just brush it; your toes should be pointing slightly outward and your feet should be flat on the floor; lower your hips and grasp the barbell at about shoulder-width, palms toward your body, arms straight; your back should be straight and your buttocks low.
Action:    On two counts:
1  Keeping your feet flat on the floor, your back and arms straight throughout the exercise, straighten up so that you are fully erect and the barbell rests at the hang;
2  Return to starting position and repeat.

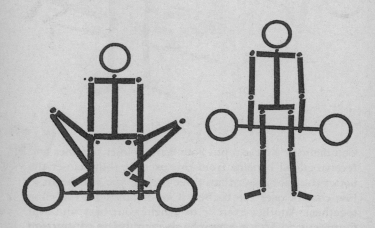

## 2 *Back Hyperextension*

**Weights:** Quite light.
**Starting Position:** Lie flat on your stomach on a bench so that the bench supports your legs as far as your hips; have an assistant hold your feet down.
**Action:** On two counts:

1 Holding the barbell behind your head (when you first start this exercise do not use more than 5 to 10 pounds), arch up as high as you can;
2 Drop below level of bench and repeat.

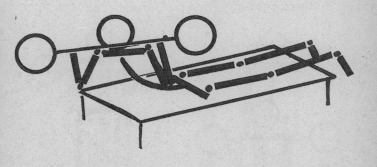

**Comments:** This movement gives complete contraction exercise to your lower back muscles.

**EXERCISES FOR THE ARM MUSCLES** (*Biceps and forearm*)

1  *Arm Curl*

Weights:  Average.

Starting Position:  Start with the barbell at the hang position; your hands should be about shoulder-width apart and your palms should be away from your body; stand comfortably with your feet about twelves inches apart.

Action:  On two counts:

1  Keeping your head up and forward, and your body erect, "curl" the weight to your chest by folding your forearms against your upper arms; keep your elbows to your sides throughout the exercise;

2  Return to starting position and repeat.

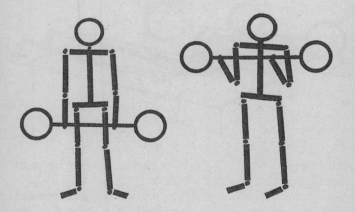

Comments:  Try to restrict all action to your arms. You can do the same exercise with your palms toward your body but you should use lighter weights.

## 2 Wrist Curl

**Weights:** Slightly lighter than average.
**Starting Position:** Sit on a bench; grasp the barbell with your hands about twelve inches apart and your palms up; support your forearms as far as your wrists by resting them on your thighs.
**Action:** On two counts:

1  Raise the barbell as far as your wrist mobility allows, working the wrist through its full range of motion;
2  Allow the barbell to roll down in your fingers as far as you safely can, and repeat.

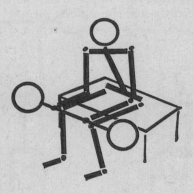

**Comments:** You can perform the same exercise with your palms in the down position.

Another variation of the Wrist Curl is to load only one end of a barbell and hold it at your side by one hand at the unloaded end of the bar. Then raise and lower the weight through the full range of your wrist mobility. Your forearm should stay stationary during this exercise. The same exercise can be done with the weighted end of the barbell extending toward the rear.

EXERCISES FOR THE SHOULDERS AND TRICEPS

1  *Military Press*

Weights:   Average.
Starting Position:   Start with the barbell at chest level;
your hands should be shoulder-width apart, palms away
from your body (at the chest position); feet should be about
twelve inches apart.
Action:   On two counts:
1  Raise the barbell to full-arm extension overhead; your
   arms should lock at the top of your motion;
2  Return to starting position and repeat.

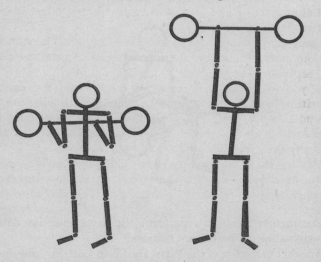

Comments:   This exercise is also excellent for developing
neck muscles.
A variation is to position your hands on the barbell a
greater distance apart than shoulder-width. Another is to
lower the barbell to the shoulders (behind the head) on
count #2.

## 2 *Bench Press* (Flat and inclined)

Weights: Average to heavier than average.
Starting Position: Lie flat on your back on a bench, with your legs straddling the bench and your feet flat on the floor; be sure that your entire upper body is supported by the bench. With your arms fully extended to the locked position directly above your head, have a partner hand you the barbell.
Action: On two counts:
1 Lower the bar to your chest;
2 Press the barbell up to the starting position, and repeat.

Comments: You can perform this exercise with your hands at shoulder-width apart, quite close together (about twelve inches), or wide apart.
Keep your elbows close to your sides to get full benefits in your arms. If you want to emphasize your pectoral muscles, keep your elbows wide.
If you do not have a partner, you can start this movement with the barbell resting on your thighs. With a leg thrust and arm lift, pull the barbell up and along your body to the chest position, press it fully overhead, and you are ready to follow the exercise as described above.
A much more strenuous version of this exercise is to raise the head end of your bench several inches. This gives even more work to your pectoral muscles. You can raise the incline of the bench as high as you like, within reason.

### EXERCISES FOR THE CHEST MUSCLES

## 1 *Pullover*

Weights: Much lighter than average.
Starting Position: Lie flat on your back on a mat; with the barbell on the floor behind your head, position your hands at shoulder-width apart; arms should be fully extended behind your head.

Action:   On two counts:
1  Without bending your elbows, arc the barbell to a
   point directly over your chest, exhaling as you raise
   the weight;
2  Return to starting position and repeat.

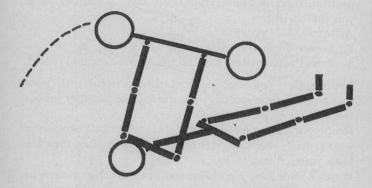

Comments:   You should use a light weight so you can
concentrate on the correct and vigorous breathing which
must accompany this exercise. When you first start practicing this exercise, the weight of the bar alone will be
enough.
Be sure to inhale fully at the start of count #1.
Another exercise which benefits your chest muscles is the
Bench Press, particularly when done with an inclined
bench.

2  *Bent-arm Lateral Raise Lying* (Dumbbell exercise)

Weights:   Less than half average weight.
Starting Position:   Lie flat on your back on a bench;
with a dumbbell in each hand, start with your arms
slightly bent at the elbow and directly over your chest.

Action:   On two counts:

1  Lower the weights in arcs — one to each side — to the
full stretch of your pectoral muscles; this action must
be accompanied by inhaling forcefully;

2  Return to starting position as you exhale, and repeat.

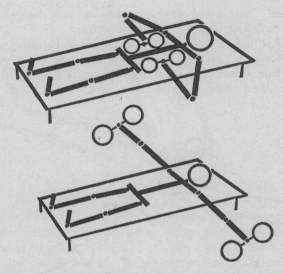

Comments:   The more you bend your elbows, within
reason, the more benefits your pectoral muscles will receive
— but be careful of too much weight. You should start
with only 5 to 10 pounds and add weight even more
gradually than usual.

This exercise can also be done from the standing position.
Lean forward from the hips so that the upper body is horizontal with the floor. Start with the dumbbells at the hang
position and your arms about twelve inches apart.

With a sweeping motion, arc the dumbbells up and to
the side to the full height of your pectoral stretch, then
return to starting position and repeat.

### 3  Bent-arm Pullover

Weights:  Lighter than average.

Starting Position:    Lie flat on your back, holding the barbell straight over your chest, with your arms locked; your hands should be about shoulder-width apart, palms toward your feet.

Action:   The action of this exercise is just the reverse from the regular pullover. On two counts:

1  Inhaling forcefully, lower the barbell by bending your elbows and arching it to a point behind your head;

2  While exhaling, return to starting position with a similar arching motion, and repeat.

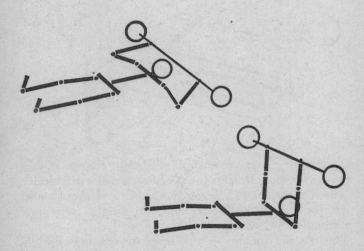

**EXERCISES FOR THE TRUNK MUSCLES** (*Lateral and abdominal*)

### 1  Side Twister

Weights:  Lighter than average.

**Starting Position:** Start with a lightly weighted barbell across your shoulders, behind your head; your feet should be about twelve inches apart; your hands should be slightly wider apart than shoulder-width, palms away from the body.

**Action:** On four counts:

1 Using only a motion to stretch the lateral trunk muscles on the left side of your body, lean or "twist" your body to the right as far as you can;
2 Return to starting position;
3 Repeat the twist action to your left;
4 Return to starting position and repeat.

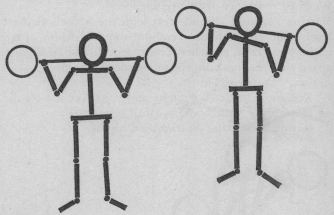

**2 Sit-ups**

**Weights:** Much lighter than average.

**Starting Position:** The conventional starting position for a sit-up calisthenic; with your hands about shoulder-width apart; palms away from the body, hold a lightly weighted barbell behind your head.

**Action:** On two counts:

1 Raise your body in a conventional Sit-up;
2 Return to starting position and repeat.

Comments: You can increase the difficulty of this exercise by raising the *foot* end of your bench. Do not raise it too high, though, or you run the risk of sliding.

We suggest that you should not use more than the weight of the barbell or at most 5 pounds of weight when you first start practicing this movement. Then add weights with great caution.

### EXERCISES FOR THE THIGHS AND HIPS

### 1  *Front Squat*

Weights: Heavier than average.

Starting Position: Stand erect with the barbell at chest level; your hands should be about shoulder-width apart, palms away from your body; your feet should be slightly apart, with the toes pointing outward at an angle.

Action: On two counts:

1 Keeping your back straight and your feet flat on the floor, lower your body to a full squat;
2 Return to starting position and repeat.

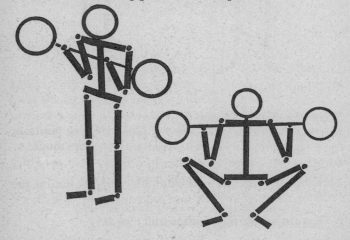

Comments: This exercise gives excellent stretching to your thigh extensors, particularly near the knees.

Variations of this exercise include Partial Knee Bends, Full Knee Bends, and Straddle Knee Bends.

With the Full Knee Bend (feet together, toes at an angle), you rise on your toes as you drop into a full squat. This not only gives additional stretching to your thigh extensors, it is also good for developing balance.

With the Straddle Knee Bend, you straddle the weight and raise it until the barbell is just under your crotch. You then perform Partial Knee Bends.

The squat is one of the most fundamental weight-training movements. You will note that we include it in each of the exercise groups we recommend.

Some people have even used squats (Full Knee Bends in particular) as a minimal, but relatively complete, weight-training workout. Not only is this an excellent exercise, but it benefits virtually the entire body so it serves as a warm-up, too. *This is the one instance where it is perfectly all right to practice weight training on a daily basis providing you do not work with extremely heavy weights.*


## 2  Shoulder Squats

Weights:   Much heavier than average.

Starting Position:   This exercise is precisely the same as the Front Squat, except that you rest the barbell on your shoulders behind your head. For the sake of convenince, you can have a partner hand you the barbell in position, or you can lift the barbell from a shoulder-high stand.

Action:   On two counts:

1  Keeping your back straight and your feet flat on the floor, lower your body to a full squat;

2  Return to starting position and repeat.

Comments:   With the exception of the Straddle Knee
Bend, you can use the same variations of the Front Squat
for this exercise.

Another variation of the modest but worth-while "one-
exercise" approach we mentioned under Front Squats, is
to perform Shoulder Squats with a press from behind the
neck after completing each repetition (*i.e.*, from standing
position). This is rather strenuous if you use fairly heavy
weights and do the normal number of repetitions. It should
be done only by itself after calisthenics and a weight training warm-up.

(Anyone who can perform three sets of 7 to 10 repetitions
each, using 75 to 100 pounds in this exercise, is above
normal in strength.)

### 3   *Leg Curl* (Leg weights)

Weights:   5 to 10 pounds, or less.

Starting Position:   This exercise may be done either lying
or standing; it involves special sandals which will accommodate a short bar and weights.

For the Leg Curl (Lying), lie flat on your stomach on a
bench; your legs should be fully extended and together.

Action:   On two counts:

1   Either individually or together, curl your leg as far
as possible and try to touch your buttocks;

2   Return to starting position, and repeat.

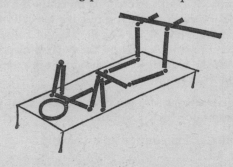

Comments: You will get increased benefits from this exercise if you incline the head of your bench. If the angle is too steep, you may not be able to touch your buttocks, but you should curl your legs up as far as you can. Note that for progressive strengthening, you can add weights, incline the board, or both.

To perform the Leg Curl (Standing), stand on one leg on a box, keeping your balance by holding to a door frame or mounted hand grip. Be sure that the foot with the sandal clears the floor.

To perform the exercise, simply curl your leg to maximum contraction. Then switch feet and repeat the series.

### 4 Rear Squats

Weights: Much heavier than average.
Starting Position: For this exercise, you will need a low rack which supports the barbell a few inches off the floor.

Start at the squat position, with your feet about twelve inches apart and your heels raised at least two inches off the floor by a board; grasp the barbell behind your body with your hands somewhat farther apart than shoulder-width, palms away from the body.
Action: On two counts:
1 Keeping the back straight, rise to an erect position;
2 Return to starting position and repeat.

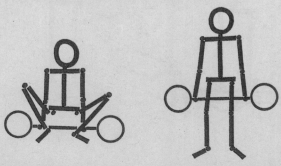

Comments:    This exercise is sometimes referred to as the
"Rack Lift." Note that the weight does not hang free at the
squat position; you must hold it a few inches off the floor
with your arms.

**EXERCISES FOR THE CALF MUSCLES**

### 1  *Rise-on-toes*

Weights:    Much heavier than average.
Starting Position:    Take the barbell from a shoulder
rack, or have an assistant place it in position; start with the
barbell across your shoulders at the back of your neck;
your hands should be farther apart than shoulder-width,
with the palms away from the body; the balls of your feet
should be supported by a two-inch board so that you start
the exercise with your heels about two inches lower than
your toes.
Action:    On two counts:
1   Rise on your toes as high as you can;
2   Return to starting position.

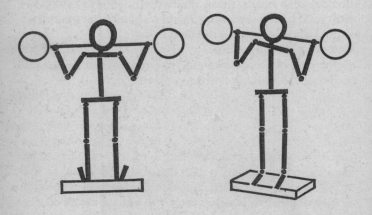

Comments: Your calf muscles are difficult to develop because they are already so strong from walking — even in a person who is relatively inactive. Therefore you must use heavier weights than you normally would in other exercises. For best results, you should do repetitions in three different ways — one with your toes pointing slightly inward; one with the toes pointing slightly outward; and one with the toes straight ahead.

## 2 *Vertical Jumping*

Weights: Lighter than average.
Starting Position: Place a fairly light barbell on your shoulders, behind your head; your hands should be slightly wider apart than shoulder-width, palms away from your body.
Action: On two counts:
1 Jump into the air as high as you can, developing as much spring as you can from your calf muscles, and as little as possible from your thigh muscles;
2 Return to starting position and repeat.

Comments: It is a good idea to place a folded towel or pad across your shoulders or wrap it around the barbell so that you won't bruise your backbone.
You should do twice as many repetitions of this exercise as you would normally do for others because it is so difficult to develop the calf muscles.
A variation of this exercise is the Straddle Hop. Rather than jump into the air, you jump to a straddle position on count #1. Try not to bend your knees during this exercise — *i.e.*, bounce on your toes, keeping your legs as straight as possible. In this exercise, padding is even more important than in vertical jumping because of the tendency of the barbell to bounce around. Hold the bar low on your shoulders so that the trapezius muscle will keep pressure off the spine.

# 8

## ISOMETRICS

Although isometrics is a relatively recent development, its effectiveness in building strength has been thoroughly tested and proved throughout the NFL. Through isometrics you can develop explosive power and strength with little effort and over a relatively short period of time.

Blanton Collier, coach of the Cleveland Browns, tells a story about one of his players who uses isometrics:

"Mike Lucci, one of our linebackers, does his isometrics in his apartment. His shoulders have become so strong that he's actually widened the door frames in his living room an inch and a half."

You can gain in strength by using isometrics with your muscles in any position. But research has shown that you will derive the greatest benefits by practicing isometric contractions while your muscles are slightly shorter than they are in their normal resting positions.

Clint Houy, trainer of the Dallas Cowboys, has this to say about the strength-building powers of isometrics:

"If an average person follows a well-rounded program of

isometrics faithfully, he can expect a definite increase in strength every week, after the first seven days of exercise. Any normal man can greatly increase his strength over a 20-week period, although he won't really 'feel' the effects for a week or so after he starts."

Below you will find three groups of isometric exercises: BASIC, ADVANCED, and INTENSIVE.

Neither the BASIC nor ADVANCED group requires any equipment; the INTENSIVE group requires a power rack* and bench.

* Each counts as two exercises.

## The BASIC Group

Included are two warm-ups and six exercises, which will provide a good strengthening program for your body muscles. For these exercises (which do not involve any equipment) we suggest a moderate length of contraction time: 6 to 9 seconds.

† See instructions on building a power rack, at the end of this chapter.

## The ADVANCED Group

Included are two warm-ups and ten exercises which will build up the strength of your entire body. These exercises do not involve any special equipment. We suggest a longer contraction time: 6 to 11 seconds.

* Each counts as two exercises.

## The INTENSIVE Group

These exercises — two warm-ups and ten isometrics — require a power rack and a sturdy bench. We recommend a contraction time from 6 to 13 seconds.

* Each counts as two exercises.

## How To Perform Isometric Exercises

Isometrics is a perfectly safe method of building strength, if properly performed. *Never try to do an isometric exercise without becoming thoroughly familiar with the following rules.*

YOU CAN EXERCISE EVERY DAY   Because isometric exercises cause little fatigue, you can practice them every day. But always rest a few seconds between exercises. If both isometrics and weight training are included in your program, perform the weight training first.

*Optional:*   A moderate but perfectly good training program can involve isometrics on an every-other-day basis. Simply perform calisthenics one day, and two warm-up exercises and isometrics the next day.

(*Caution:*   We strongly recommend that nobody under the age of 13 years engage in isometrics. For they are still going through too many bodily changes to engage in anything but calisthenics and a very mild weight-training program.)

**ALWAYS COMBINE CALISTHENICS WITH ISOMETRICS**  We suggest two warm-up calisthenics as a minimum before performing isometrics. Normally, you should perform a group of calisthenics prior to isometrics.

Dr. Theodore Fox, team physician for the Chicago Bears, explains how calisthenics "balance" the results of isometrics:

"If muscles are to remain supple, isometrics must be accompanied by calisthenics to tone and flex the muscles and keep them limber. Otherwise, muscles would never get the *stretching* they need and eventually would lose their flexibility."

**LEARN TO RELAX ANTAGONISTIC MUSCLES**  Ordinarily, when you flex a group of muscles or use them in bodily movement, the "antagonistic" group of extensors relaxes. This is a natural result of good coordination between muscles and nerves.

When you do an isometric exercise, however, there is a tendency to tighten your triceps as well as your biceps, for example. Try to avoid this by concentrating on relaxing your triceps while creating maximum tension in your biceps. Otherwise you won't get the full benefit of the contraction on your biceps alone.

**EASE IN AND OUT OF CONTRACTIONS**  You should spend the first two seconds of an isometric contraction *gradually increasing* your muscular force. Then, after holding a maximum contraction, *gradually decrease* the force during the final two seconds.

As an example: If you use a 7-second contraction, you will actually flex your muscles at maximum strength for only three seconds; but you will still get plenty of benefit from the exercise.

"Easing in and out" of a contraction acts as a safety factor by preventing a sudden strain on your muscles.

HOW LONG TO HOLD A CONTRACTION   When you start practicing isometrics, use a short contraction period. Increase the time of the contraction by adding one second at a time to the period of maximum contraction, keeping the "easing in and out" time of 2 seconds at the start and end of the exercise.

*Do not get overly ambitious and try to increase your "holding time" too quickly*. You should practice an exercise at lease two weeks before increasing the hold time by one second.

You must realize that there is a limit to how long you can maintain maximum tension on a muscle. After a certain length of time (it varies with the individual) the muscles simply can't sustain the effort, and the contraction starts to "drain away."

*We strongly recommend that you do not try to maintain a maximum contraction for longer than 9 seconds* (a 13-second hold which includes a 2-second ease-in and ease-off).

If you try to hold a contraction longer than your muscular capability, you're wasting your time. The benefits from isometrics depend on maximum contraction.

BREATHE PROPERLY   It is perfectly all right to hold your breath while holding a maximum contraction — but never to the point where you start feeling light-headed or dizzy.

You should *never* hold your breath longer than 9 seconds.

The proper way to breathe is to take a deep breath at the start of an exercise, hold it for a few seconds, and exhale slowly. (If you need more than one breath for a relatively long contraction, repeat the process.)

DON'T PERFORM TOO MANY EXERCISES   Since isometric exercises are so easy to perform, many people are tempted to go through their routine more than once a day. But do not yield to this temptation. *Performing an isometric more than once won't do you any more good than a single maxi-mum contraction.*

USE SPECIAL ISOMETRICS IF YOU WISH    If you want to de-velop particular muscles — because they are underdevel-oped or you need them for a sport — go ahead and include special isometrics in your program.* But don't perform more than a total of 10 isometrics in your program.

* Special exercises will be described in the following chapter.

## Isometric Exercises (No Equipment Needed)

In the exercises below, we do not draw a distinction be-tween a BASIC and an ADVANCED isometric. The differ-ence between them is determined only by how long a contraction is held.

1   *Chest Expansion* (Pectoral muscles)

Action:    Stand a few inches from one side of a door frame; take up a comfortable stance with your feet about six to eight inches apart; place one hand on each side of the door frame, palms flat and toward each other; inhale fully and squeeze to maximum contraction, as you exhale slowly.

2   *Shoulder Contraction* (Shoulders, upper back muscles)

Action:    Stand in a doorway about three feet wide, with one hand on each side of the door frame and at shoulder height or a little higher; palms should be flat against the frame and away from your body; inhale fully and push outward to maximum contraction as you exhale slowly. This exercise is excellent for removing fat from the upper arms.

3   *Trunk Contraction* (Lateral trunk, abdominal, arm, and shoulder muscles)

Action: Take up a semi-crouch position, knees slightly bent and apart, feet about shoulder-width apart; place hands on legs slightly above the knees. Inhale fully and push down to maximum contraction as you exhale slowly. (Note that your body itself acts as the immovable object in this exercise.)

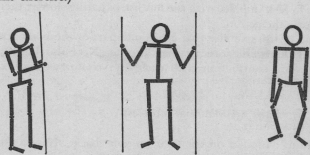

4 *Leg Contraction* (Leg, hip, and stomach muscles)

Action: Stand flush against one side of a doorway that is about three feet wide; raise one leg so that your foot is against the opposite side of the door frame and about belt high. Inhale fully and push against the door frame to maximum contraction with your leg as you exhale slowly. Then repeat with the other leg.

Note that one isometric contraction with each leg counts as two isometric exercises.

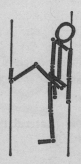

5  *Arm Contraction*  (Primarily biceps and forearm
   muscles)

Action:    Stand erect, feet about shoulder-width apart;
place left fist in right hand, keeping forearms parallel to
the floor; inhale fully and try to raise the right hand while
you hold it in place with the left fist, exhaling slowly; then
reverse the action.
Note in this exercise that again one part of the body acts
as an immovable force against the other. Note also that one
isometric contraction with each arm counts as two exercises.

6  *Leg Raise*  (Abdominal muscles)

Action:   Lie flat on the floor on your back, arms to the
sides; lift legs about one foot off the floor and hold stationary for the duration of the isometric hold period.
Note that technically this is not a true isometric. Never-
theless, with the weight of your legs acting as a force against
your abdominal muscles, this is an excellent exercise for
building strength. It is also good for eliminating excess
weight around the middle.

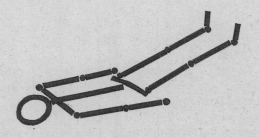

7 *Neck Hold* (Neck muscles)

Action: Clasp your fingers behind your neck. Inhale fully and force your head back against your clasped hands to maximum contraction, as you exhale slowly.
This exercise is excellent for posture improvement.

8 *Neck Contraction* (Neck muscles)

Action (for muscles at the front of the neck): Fold a towel several times so that it makes a thick pad; place the folded towel against a door frame and hold it in place with your forehead. Your feet should be slightly apart and about a foot from the frame. Place one hand on each side of the door frame for balance. Inhale fully and press with your head against the door frame to maximum contraction, exhaling slowly.

Action (for muscles at the back of the neck): Hold towel in place with the back of your head as you stand in the door frame; reach back with your hands, one on each side of the door frame, for balance. Inhale fully and press back with your head against the door frame to maximum contraction, exhaling slowly.
Note that this exercise is excellent for posture improvement.

## Isometric Exercises
## (Power Rack and Bench Needed)

Do at least two warm-ups — one of them a calisthenic (Jumping Jack, Shadow Boxing, or Running in Place), the other, a Bar Hang.*

* See chapter on CALISTHENICS for instructions on how to perform these exercises.

Using one of the three warm-up calisthenics we suggest above is certainly not a "must." Any toe touch, squatting, or stretching calisthenic which gives vigorous stretching and flexing to your entire body makes a perfectly good warm-up.

1   *Shoulder Shrug* (Shoulder muscles; also upper trapezius muscles of back and neck)

Bar height:   At the same height your hands naturally fall when you are standing erect, arms fully extended at your sides; grasp the bar with your hands at shoulder-width apart.
Action:Inhale fully and pull up on the bar to maximum contraction by shrugging your shoulders, while exhaling slowly.

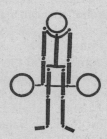

2   *Rise-on-toes— Seated* (Calf muscles)

Bar height:   Sit on a padded bench. Place a two-foot long 2-by-4 under your toes and adjust the bar so that it is just above your knees; fold a towel over so that it becomes a thick pad and place it on top of your knees to protect them; let your arms hang fully to your sides.
Action:   Inhale fully and push up to full contraction against the bar with your knees by raising your heels, while exhaling slowly. One day do this exercise with the toes pointing out; the next day, pointing in; the following day, pointing straight ahead.

Comments:   The same exercise can be done from a standing position by adjusting the bar so that it rests across your shoulder muscles; feet should be flat on the floor and about twelve inches apart; rise on your toes as in the seated position. This exercise also develops your neck and back muscles as well as the calf muscles.

You may have to back up a little and then lean forward slightly, keeping your back straight, in order to get a better push. Also, you may want to use a folded towel between your shoulders and the bar as a pad.

3 *Military Press* (Triceps, shoulder, neck, back, abdominal, and leg muscles)

Bar height:   About two inches above your head.

Action:   Stand directly under the bar; looking straight ahead, grasp the bar with your hands about shoulder-width apart, palms away from your body; inhale fully and push up with your arm, shoulder, leg, hip, and back muscles to maximum contraction, while exhaling slowly.

4 *Leg Curl* (Flexor or hamstring muscles at the backs of upper legs)

Bar height:   For this exercise, lie on your stomach on a bench; adjust the bar so that you can flex your legs only about halfway between the horizontal and the vertical, and your heels touch the bar. You may want to fold a towel into a pad and place it under your knees.

Action:   Grasping the bench with your hands, and hooking your heels against the bar, inhale fully and flex or "curl" your legs to maximum contraction, trying to pull the bar toward you, while exhaling slowly.

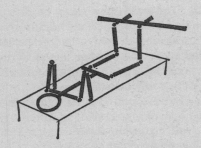

Comments:   This exercise helps develop quickness in starting and running.

An alternate position for the exercise is to raise the bar so that your heels just meet it when your legs are curled to the vertical position. The action for the exercise is exactly the same as for that above.

5   *Bench Press* (Arm, shoulder, and chest muscles)

Bar height:   Lie on a bench or mat under the bar so that it is directly above your shoulders; place the bar at a height which is just short of maximum extension of your arms.

Action:   Inhale fully, and push up to maximum contraction against the bar, while exhaling slowly.

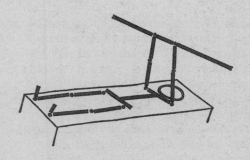

6   *Leg Press* (Leg muscles)

Bar height:   Lie on your back on a bench, with your hips
directly under the bar, your arms to your sides and palms
flat (or you can grasp the bench); adjust the height of the
bar so that when your raised feet touch it, your knees are
partially flexed and just short of maximum extension as in
the diagram; keep your pelvis flat on the bench to avoid
undue strain on your back, and hold your head up so that
your chin is near your chest.
Action:   Inhale fully, and push up to maximum contraction against the bar, while exhaling slowly.
Comments:   A strong professional football player can
exert as much as a ton of force in this exercise.

7   *Arm Curl* (Biceps and forearm muscles)
Bar height:   Place bar at a height slightly below the point
where your elbow falls when you are standing erect; flex
your arms so that your forearms are horizontal and your
wrists are under the bar and about shoulder-width apart.
Action:   Inhale fully, and pull up to maximum contraction, while exhaling slowly.

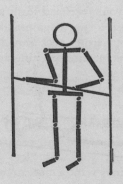

8 *High Press* (Arm, back, and shoulder muscles)

Bar height:   Set the bar slightly lower than your maximum reach when you stretch your arms overhead.
Action:   Grasping the bar with your hands about shoulder-width apart, inhale fully, and push up to maximum contraction with your arm, back, hip, and leg muscles, while exhaling slowly; look straight ahead during the exercise.

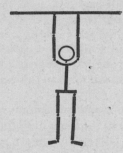

9 *Neck Contraction* (Neck muscles)

Bar height:   Level with your eyes.
Action:   Fold a towel so that it makes a thick pad, and place it between your forehead and the bar; standing erect, feet about shoulder-width apart, lean slightly forward from the waist so that your forehead leans against the bar; inhale fully, and push forward against the bar to maximum contraction of your front neck muscles, while exhaling slowly. Repeat the exercise, pushing against the bar with the back of your head.
Comments:   This exercise counts as two isometrics.

## How To Measure Your Progress

There is no way to measure your progress using isometrics alone. Before long, you will "feel" your increase in strength, but you may want a more accurate measure.

Unless you purchase special equipment, lifting weights is the only way to determine progress — by measuring before you start your isometrics program, and then at regular intervals. If you decide to follow this procedure, we suggest you read the chapter on weight training. You should not approach this chapter in a casual fashion. You should read it just as though you were going to undertake a full weight-training program on a regular basis. Practice the necessary motions, and observe all rules concerning technique, precautions, warm-up, resting periods, etc.

All testing exercises recommended involve a barbell:

> Arm Curl
> Upright Rowing
> Bench Press
> Rowing Motion
> Military Press

There five exercises will measure primarily the development of your arm, back, shoulder, abdominal, and chest muscles. Trying to measure the development of your leg muscles is impractical. In the first place, your leg muscles are the most powerful in your body. Providing you follow a well-rounded group of isometric exercises, your legs will develop in rough proportion to your other muscles, although they won't increase in strength by as great a percentage. Secondly, measuring the increase in strength of your leg muscles would probably involve using heavier weights than you should.

Before starting isometrics training, perform each test exercise, using enough weight so that your muscles are just beginning to tire after 6 to 8 repetitions.

On future tests, see how many additional repetitions you can do easily and without tiring. As soon as your muscles begin to show signs of tiring (you will feel it), consider this to be the end of the test for the exercise. Do not make this a competitive thing; it is a test. If you try to do more repetitions than you really can perform easily, you are just kidding yourself.

As soon as you can perform 15 to 20 repetitions of an exercise, add 20 pounds to the barbell for future tests.

## How To Build a Power Rack

Mount two sturdy timbers upright, about three to four feet apart (we prefer a three-foot distance between uprights). Then drill holes in each timber at various levels (pairs of holes — one on each timber — must be at the same level, of course); then slip a solid steel bar through holes at whatever level you want to practice isometrics.

You can mount the upright timbers one of two ways:

1  Bolt the tops securely to the overhead crosspieces of a garage or cellar ceiling; then anchor the bottoms in position by driving wedges between the foot of each timber and the floor.

2  Sink the timbers in holes outdoors (about 18 inches deep), and pour concrete around them.

The timbers should be at least 4-by-6, and preferably 4-by-12. You will want well-preserved timbers that are about ten feet tall. If you are mounting them outdoors, it is a good idea to paint them with some kind of wood preservative as a protection against the weather.

Drill pairs of holes — one in each support — at the same height. If you do not know how to mark off the timbers to be sure your pairs of holes will be level, check with a carpenter. The diameter of your holes should be slightly larger than the diameter of your steel bar.

Drill holes from a point three inches from the ground to a point high enough so that your feet won't touch the ground when you hang from the bar. Be sure the centers of the holes you drill will be at least three inches from the nearest timber edge.

If you use a 4-by-6, drill holes at four-inch intervals. If you use a 4-by-12, stagger the holes so that you have an adjustment every three inches as shown below. Do not try to space your holes any closer; it is perfectly possible for an extremely strong man to rip the bar from one hole to another if they are set closer than the distance we recommend. This, of course, could lead to injury.

Use a solid steel bar — a weight-training bar will do nicely — not a hollow pipe, you may very well bend a pipe.

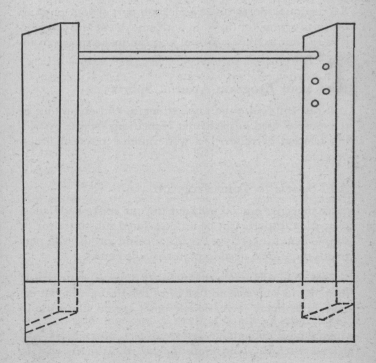

# 9

## SPORTS

Recreational sports can be a pleasant part of your physical fitness program, for they add both enjoyment and competition to your exercise routine. You can make sports an integral part of your program in one of two ways:

### Plan Your Program Around Sports

You can emphasize the tone, strength, and endurance of the muscles used in particular recreational sports by adding selected exercises to a well-rounded physical fitness program.

### Add Sports to Your Program

Since they give a good workout to your entire body, most recreational sports can be an occasional substitute for or supplement to exercises. For instance, on any day you play tennis there is no need to perform calisthenics.

Providing you match the intensity of your participation in sports to your age and physical condition, you can engage in as many recreational sports as you like without endangering your health.

To the "weekend athlete," however, recreational sports can be a great danger. The man who doesn't keep himself

154

in condition, yet occasionally participates in a marathon day of tennis, handball, or golf, is risking not only his health, but his life.

## The Common Recreational Sports

In the next few pages we analyze each of the common recreational sports — golf, tennis, handball, swimming, bowling, and skiing — in terms of the particular muscles each involves. Each sport requires good general body tone, good general coordination, and strength in certain muscles. To build up these muscles, simply perform appropriate calisthenic, isometric or weight-training exercises which increase their tone, strength, and endurance.

In this chapter, we describe several special exercises which you may want to add to your program. For your convenience, they are arranged by muscle groups.

Bill McPeak, coach of the Washington Redskins, tells how Johnny Sample used a "special exercise" to improve his play as a defensive halfback.

"In Johnny's position, strong hand and forearm muscles are a great help in making open field tackles, where you can't always hit a man head-on, but have to grab one of his limbs or part of his uniform.

"Johnny started squeezing a rubber ball about two-thirds of his waking hours. It was funny at first. But when other players saw how tremendously strong his hand and forearm muscles became, they stopped laughing.

"Now six or seven of our players have made squeezing a rubber ball a regular habit. They all report that the strength of their grip was greatly increased."

*A note of caution:* Never do just a few calisthenics, isometrics, or weight-training exercises to benefit *only* the primary muscles you need for a sport. Since each recreational sport involves your entire body, you should always follow a group of exercises which give benefits to all the muscles in your body. The special exercises we suggest in this chapter are to help you put an emphasis on key muscles. *This does not mean that you should ignore the development of the rest of your body.*

To help you determine which muscles will need attention to improve your performance in a sport, we have analyzed each sport below. Following this section, we describe special exercises which you may find useful.

GOLF   Golf benefits the tone of many of your muscles because so much walking and movement is involved. The game requires particular strength in your back, shoulder, arm, and wrist muscles.

TENNIS   This sport gives an excellent workout to your entire body. It requires good wind endurance as well as good leg endurance, plus strength in your back, arm, shoulder, and particularly wrist muscles.

HANDBALL   Like tennis, handball is an excellent exercise in itself for wind endurance, leg endurance, and general body tone. But if you want to play the game very well, you will probably want exceptional wind and leg endurance. The sport also requires strong leg, arm, shoulder, and back muscles.

SWIMMING   This sport involves all the muscles of your body. To excel, you will need good endurance in your entire body, plus particular strength and endurance in your leg, arm, and shoulder muscles.

SKIING  Skiing, too, brings all the muscles of your body into play. You will need particularly good endurance and strength in your leg, arm, and shoulder muscles.

BOWLING  To develop great skill in this sport, you will want to build up the strength of your arm, wrist, and shoulder muscles.

## Exercises To Improve Performance

If you are interested in improving your ability in any sport, we suggest you follow a well-balanced group of appropriate exercises — supplemented by additional exercises to benefit the key muscles you need to excel in that sport.

SPECIAL EXERCISES FOR SPORTS

*Wind Endurance*  Add a modified version of roadwork or Wind Sprints to your regular calisthenics exercises.

*Leg Muscles* (Strength and endurance)

1  Add Rope Skipping to your regular calisthenics (see pages 98-99).
2  Perform the Scissors calisthenic using light weights attached to your feet (see page 84).
3  Perform 30 to 50 repetitions of the following exercise each day:
Stand beside an 18-inch bench; step up onto the bench and return to the floor — first with one leg and then the other; each time, come to a full stop on the bench and when you return to the floor; otherwise you will lose part of the benefits of this exercise through body momentum.
This exercise is excellent for building up the strength and endurance of your leg muscles, particularly those around the knee. Note that this is really

a weight-training exercise because your legs work
against the resistance of your body weight.

4   A good weight-training exercise to build up strength
and endurance of your leg muscles is to sit on a table,
with your weight supported as far as your knee, and
your lower legs hanging free; attach light weights to
your legs, and practice lifting your lower legs to full
extension — first one leg and then the other; we
suggest 10 to 20 repetitions of this exercise with each
leg, using light weights.

Dale Meinert, linebacker for the St. Louis Cardinals, used
this exercise to build up the strength of the muscles
around his knee after a serious injury.

Danny Villanueva, place-kicking specialist for the Los
Angeles Rams, greatly increased the power of his kicking
leg by using the same principle of exercise. Rather than
sit on a table, he took the exercise one step further: he
attached small weights to his kicking leg and then practiced kicks — again and again.

*Note:*   This exercise, like many others in this book, can
be used or adapted to rehabilitation exercises. We suggest
that you never try to do this without first consulting your
physician.

*Wrist and Forearm Muscles*  (Strength)
1   The Wrist Curl and its many variations are excellent exercises for wrist and forearm muscles (see
page 123).
2   The Golfer's Roll is an improvised version of a Wrist
Curl.
Simply attach one end of a heavy cord securely to a
five- to ten-pound weight; attach the other end to the
center of a two-foot round bar (such as a broom handle); be sure to affix the cord to the round bar so that

it will not slip (you may want to drill a hole through the center).

Sit on a stool or bench with your forearms supported as far as the wrist by your thighs; grip the bar with your hands about six inches apart and the weight suspended between your legs; roll the bar so that the cord wraps around it, lifting up the weight.

Perform this exercise first with your palms up, then with them down — at least ten times each way. Be sure to work your wrists throughout their full range of motion while rolling up the weight.

3   Another excellent exercise to improve the strength of your grip, wrist, and forearm muscles, is to squeeze a tennis ball or a spring tension grip at least 15 minutes a day.

*Arm and Shoulder Muscles* (Strength)

1   Any of the isometric or weight-training exercises for these muscles.

2   *Tennis Isometric:* Holding your tennis racket with a normal grip, place the tip of the racket at an angle against a wall; take a deep breath and try to push the tennis racket through the wall. (You should perform this isometric and the ones below according to the rules described in Chapter XI.)

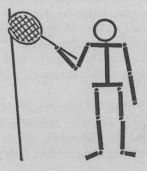

3 *Golf Isometric:* Holding your golf club with a
   normal grip, place the head of the club at an angle
   against a wall, about an inch from the floor (simulate
   addressing a ball); take a deep breath and try to push
   the head of the club through the wall.
4 *Bowling Isometric:* Select a stationary object, such as
   a radiator or heavy sofa; assume the normal position
   you would use in delivering the ball; then grip the
   radiator at that same height and try to pull it forward.

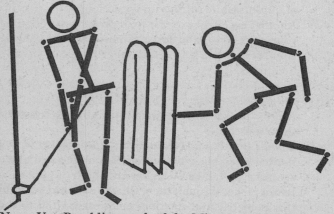

Norm Van Brocklin, coach of the Minnesota Vikings, tells
how his quarterback, Fran Tarkenton, strengthened his
throwing arm by using a special exercise:

"Fran was blessed with an exceptionally accurate throwing arm, but he needed more strength.

"To build up his arm and shoulder muscles, he practiced
his throwing motion again and again, while holding light
weights.

"To strengthen his wrist muscles, he sat on a stool, held
a light weight in his hand, and snapped his wrist forward
in a throwing motion — again and again.

"This exercise added 15 yards to the length of Fran's
passes."

# 10

## THE HEART

Many people have an unreasonable fear that exercise is harmful to their hearts.

*Sensible exercise does not pose any danger whatever to the normal heart.*

Exercise not only stimulates the rate and force of your heartbeat, but also deepens your breathing. Both are beneficial to your state of physical fitness.

Your heart is a special kind of muscle with an incredible endurance. In just one day it pumps roughly 20 tons of blood, and, if you are under stress or engage in heavy exercise, it can pump as much as 100 tons. The work your heart does even on a normal day is equivalent to that required to lift about ten tons of ice onto a six-foot platform.

By stimulating the rate and force of your heartbeat, exercise builds up the heart's "cardiac reserve." This increased action makes the heart stronger, and capable of performing without strain in times of stress.

Everyone should undertake a program of physical fitness with caution, as we have pointed out repeatedly. Even younger men should have a complete check-up before embarking on an exercise program, or going out for a school athletic team. Anyone with a known heart condition — or physical signs indicating he may have such a condition — should consult a doctor at once, and then proceed only under medical guidance. The older a man becomes, the milder his exercises should be, simply as a matter of common sense.

But as long as you *use* your common sense about exercising (no 36 holes of golf on a hot Saturday if you haven't been exercising regularly), your physical fitness program will not only benefit your body muscles, but your heart as well.

# 11

## POSTURE

Most men are a fraction of an inch shorter than their true height, simply because they don't stand fully upright. The man with good posture stands out in any crowd. He carries his head high, and conveys an impression of confidence and optimism the moment he walks into a room.

### Poor Posture Is Easy To See

You can check your own posture very simply. Just take a good look in a mirror. Are your shoulders rounded? Is one higher than the other? Does your chest disappear into your abdomen? Does your stomach sag when you don't "suck it in"? Does your chin drop forward and hang out over your chest? Is your spine unnaturally curved? When you sit down, are you inclined to slump forward?

If your answer is "yes" to any of these questions, you should add several posture-correcting exercises* to your physical fitness program.

---

* See the end of this chapter.

## Poor Posture Is Often Related to Excess Weight

Few men have problems with excess weight until they get to their mid-thirties. Before then, any posture problems can usually be remedied by corrective exercises. It is not so simple if a man puts on excess weight as he grows older. For a "rubber tire" around his middle will prevent all the corrective exercises in the world from improving his posture.

Excess weight — usually in the form of an overhanging abdomen — pulls his spine out of shape and puts an unnatural strain on the back, neck, and stomach muscles which control posture. If the condition continues, it causes cramping of body organs, pressure on nerves, and eventually a general body fatigue. The fatigue, in turn, causes more slumping, more strain, and more pressure.

The older a man gets, the more this condition can be a direct threat to his health, causing such physical ills as constipation, dizziness, shortness of breath, and indigestion — to say nothing of aches and pains.

## Good Posture Is Vital to Physical Fitness

Good posture means that you stand, walk, and sit with a minimum amount of strain on your body. It means that your organs have room to function efficiently. You feel better and look better.

Practicing good posture — all the time — is really a mild exercise in itself. Certainly, all of us do a great deal of walking in the course of a week — even the man who sits behind a desk for eight hours a day. If you practice good posture, this will contribute to your physical fitness. If you don't, it will partially nullify the benefits you would normally receive from a physical fitness program.

## How To Improve Your Posture

*Be conscious of your posture at all times.* Practice walking correctly all the time. Your body should be erect, with your shoulders back and your back naturally arched; keep your chin up, your head high, and your stomach in.

Exercises to improve your posture are concerned primarily with improving the tone of the muscles that control your posture. Additional strength, particularly in your abdominal muscles, is also important. (If you are overweight, you must combine posture exercises with a weight-control program.)

The corrective exercises listed below are all excellent for helping you improve your posture. We suggest 5 to 10 repetitions or more for each exercise. You can easily add several of these exercises to your physical fitness program. They take very little effort and only a few minutes of time. If you want additional exercises, simply add calisthenic, weight-training, or isometric exercises that benefit your neck, back, and stomach muscles.

*Reminder:*   If you have any abnormal physical condition which causes poor posture, you should consult a doctor.

## Exercises To Improve Your Posture

1   *Abdominal Retraction* (To improve standing position)

Starting Position:   Stand erect against a wall with your heels about four inches away, but your hips, shoulders, and head touching the wall.
Action:   Flatten the lower part of your back against the wall by pulling in your abdominal muscles; holding this position, come away from the wall, keeping your weight forward on the balls of your feet; maintain this position as you walk around the room for a few seconds; then relax and repeat.

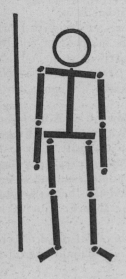

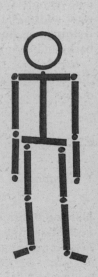

Comments:    You can also perform this exercise by lying on a bench. Simply flatten the lower part of your back against the bench by pulling in your abdominal muscles — hold it for a few seconds, then relax and repeat.

2 *Toe Rise* (To reduce unnatural but mild spinal curvature)

Starting Position: Stand erect, holding your back straight, arms to your sides, feet together. Action: Rise as high as you can on your toes, arching your arms forward and fully overhead, stretching your body as well as your arms; return to starting position and repeat.

3 *Slow Half Knee Bends* (To improve general posture)
Starting Position: Stand with your body fully erect, your feet together, and your hands clasped behind your head.
Action: Slowly drop into a half knee bend, keeping your back straight and your elbows thrust back (be sure to keep your stomach pulled in and your buttocks drawn up); return to starting position and repeat.

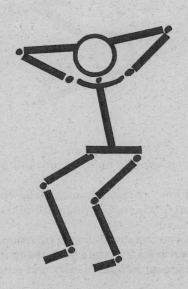

4  *Abdominal Pull* (To improve tone of your stomach
    muscles)

Starting Position:    Lie on your back, with your feet fully
extended and together, your hands clasped at the back of
your neck.
Action:    As you pull your feet up to touch your buttocks,
pull your abdomen in hard; return to starting position
and repeat.

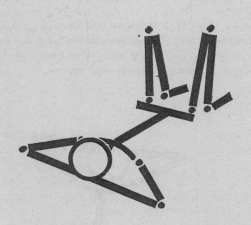

5  *Pelvic Rotations* (To improve tone of back muscles)

Starting Position:    Stand against a wall, with your heels,
shoulders, and head touching the wall; inhale and exhale
slowly and deeply.
Action:    As you exhale, pull your pelvis up in front and
down in back, using the muscles of your abdomen and
buttocks; relax and repeat.

Comments: To get the full benefits of this exercise, which forces a flattening of your lower back against the wall, do not lean your head forward.

6 *Neck Flex* (To improve tone of neck muscles)
See description of this exercise under Calesthenics (page 95).

## WEIGHT-TRAINING EXERCISES

Listed in the chapter on weight training are standard exercises which will improve the strength and endurance of your neck, abdominal, and back muscles. Any of these exercises will help improve your posture — providing they are done with regular calisthenics plus special posture-correcting calisthenics.

## ISOMETRIC EXERCISES

1 *Upper Abdominal Contraction* (Slims the waistline and benefits upper abdominal muscles)

Action: Lie flat on your back; clasping your hands behind your head, raise your upper trunk about sixteen inches off the floor and hold the position for 6 to 10 seconds.

2 *Leg Raise* (Improves abdominal sag)
See description of this under Isometrics (page 144).

3 *Neck Hold* (Strengthens neck muscles)
See description of this under Isometrics (page 145).

# 12

## WEIGHT CONTROL

Everyone should be concerned with the subject of weight control — not only *how much* weight, but *what kind* of weight, and how it is distributed throughout your body. This relates directly to your state of physical fitness.

Whether you are underweight, overweight, or of average weight, you should aim at replacing fat and flab with muscle and firm tissue. For most people this will be as simple as undertaking an intelligent physical fitness program. But if you tend to be overweight or underweight, you should take this into consideration in planning your physical fitness program.

*(Important: People with extreme cases of obesity, or with glandular or hereditary problems, should never attempt a weight-control program without consulting a doctor.)*

Providing your weight problem is primarily dietary, simply adapt the following fundamental principles to your particular needs.

### Everyone Needs a Balanced Diet

Your diet must include the right kinds of food, in sufficient variety, to satisfy the replacement, growth, and energy needs of your body.

## Everyone Must Match His Food Intake to His Energy Output

During a day you burn up bodily substances that amount to about 2,000 to 3,000 calories of energy. This varies with the individual's body chemistry and amount of activity. A professional football player will burn up from 3,000 to 4,000 calories of energy per day.

If your diet supplies more energy food (calories) than you really need, your body will convert the excess to fat unless you perform the right type and amount of exercise.

If your diet supplies less energy food than you really need, your body will eventually become undernourished and underweight.

## Proper Weight Control Must Involve Exercises and Diet

The overweight man must gradually reduce his intake of food and perform increasingly strenuous exercises. Neither diet nor exercise will do the job alone. If he tries to reduce his diet without exercising, he will simply reduce his bodily fat, rather than firm up his muscles and tissues. If he tries to exercise without dieting, he is just wasting his time. It would require a 36-mile walk to work off just one pound of fat.

The underweight man proceeds very differently: he must combine an increased diet with relatively mild exercise, which keeps the body toned and builds up his muscles and tissues. If he doesn't exercise, the additional weight will turn into fat.

## Proper Weight Control Requires Self-Discipline

Since exercise tends to build up the appetite, the overweight man, in particular, must use considerable self-discipline if he really wants to make progress.

One way to fight hunger pangs is to include plenty of high-bulk, low-calorie foods in a diet (such as fruits, vegetables, and lean meats).

## Proper Nutrition Is Vital to Health

"Diet" simply refers to the food you eat. You can have a normal diet, a reduced diet ("dieting"), or an increased diet. But whatever the case, you must have a *balanced* diet, which includes sufficient amounts of five different types of substances:

1 CARBOHYDRATES    These "energy foods," such as pastries, bread, other starchy foods, cereal grains, and sweets, account for about 50 percent of the calories in a normal diet. Your body converts carbohydrates into energy or body fat.

2 FATS    These contribute roughly 25 to 30 percent of the calories in a normal diet, and include butter, cream, fatty meats, mayonnaise, etc. The body converts fats into energy, or stores them as body fat. (Fats are probably the most difficult kind of food for your system to digest.)

3 PROTEINS    These are the basic building materials of the body. They include meats, fowl, fish, milk, eggs, cheese, nuts, and whole-grain products. Proteins contain far fewer calories than carbohydrates or fats. Your body breaks down proteins into substances which it then uses to replace and build tissue.

4 VITAMINS    The normal diet contains all the vitamins necessary for healthy living: Vitamin C for body resistance to disease (found in such foods as citrus fruits, fruit juices, and tomatoes), Vitamin A to stimulate growth, etc. Vitamin supplements (capsules) are sometimes of value to certain people, particularly those in a run-down condition. Your doctor can give you good advice on this.

5 MINERALS  The average diet almost always contains ample quantities of minerals, such as calcium for your bones and teeth (milk) and iron for your blood (liver, oysters).

## How To Lose Weight

DIET  Excess fat is harmful. It places great strains on your body — your internal organs, your muscles, your heart, and your organic system.

It may be true that "everybody loves a fat man" — and disease is no exception. Excess fat is believed to be related to incidence of nonhereditary heart disease, high blood pressure, cerebral hemorrhage, and many other diseases. Overweight people are far more susceptible to heart disease than the man of normal weight, and three times as susceptible to kidney trouble.

Your goal in reducing your weight should be twofold: First, to rid yourself of excess weight; second, to replace fat with firm tissue and muscle. The procedure is to combine a reduced food intake with an exercise program of gradually increasing vigorousness. If you reduce your diet by 600 to 700 calories per day, you should lose one pound of fat a week. Your doctor can help you determine how many calories are in your present diet and can make suggestions about how fast and how far you should cut down.

*Do not make sudden changes in your diet.* A gradual decrease should take place over a period of two weeks or more. This procedure will help your body get used to the change and prevent the sharp hunger pangs that otherwise would occur. (It is dangerous to reduce your food intake too far. You may not feel the detrimental effects immediately, but in the long run your body will pay a price for your rashness.)

EXERCISE  In addition to your diet, you should start a

program of exercise, based on calisthenics and isometrics. The more strenuous the calisthenics, the better.

Obviously, a poorly conditioned overweight man should not *start* with a strenuous calisthenics program. He must build up very gradually and let his body accommodate itself to the change.

The isometrics you practice will help remove excess fat from the area where you contract your muscles. The Shoulder Contraction isometric will slim fat off your upper arms, for example.

## How To Gain Weight

DIET    *Mild exercises* combined with an *increased* but *balanced diet* will put weight on almost anyone.

But do not suddenly increase the amount of calories in your diet. Instead, build it up over a period of several weeks. Not only should you increase the amount of food you eat at mealtime, but you should "snack" between meals. Foods which are especially rich in energy are butter, cream, fatty meats, mayonnaise, cream soups, pies, custards, ice cream, and eggnoggs.

### EXERCISE

We suggest a combination of mild calisthenics and mild weight training on alternate days: One day, perform 5 to 6 repetitions of basic calisthenics; on alternate days, perform the following:

1   Mild calisthenic warm-up (pages 64-67)
2   Weight-training warm-up (3 repetitions, each phase) (pages 114-15)
3   Basic group of weight-training exercises, 5 to 6 repetitions with moderate weights (pages 105-6)

The calisthenics will keep your body limber and well-toned without a great expenditure of energy. The weight training will build up the bulk and size of your muscles, so that your added weight will take the form of muscles and firm tissue rather than fat.

## How To Control Weight (For the Average Man)

If you are neither underweight nor overweight, but are soft and flabby, you can solve your problem by undertaking any variation of Program II. Naturally, you should start with some form of Program I and gradually increase the intensity of your exercises. Since all you have to do is to convert flab into muscle, you do not need to change your diet, providing it is balanced.

Calisthenics will tone and limber your body; weight training or isometrics will help you convert fat into firm tissue.

*Reminder.    If any person is seriously underweight or overweight, or has any abnormal physical or organic condition, it is absolutely imperative for him to work closely with his doctor. We strongly urge any person who feels he should make changes in his diet to seek the advice of his physician.*

## Training Table Menus

The importance of proper eating habits is discussed under the heading "Nutrition" in the first chapter of this book.

The methods of controlling your weight by combining exercise with proper diet are covered in the chapter WEIGHT CONTROL. We learn that an overweight man should follow an exercise program which helps him lose bulk — and must eat foods which keep him strong but prevent him from gaining weight.

The underweight man should follow an exercise program which will add bulk to his body — ideally, in the form of muscle. His diet must include foods which encourage his body to add weight. `

But *any* balanced diet — whether for the man who is too fat, too thin, or "just right" — must include five basic ingredients in order to offer proper nutrition: carbohydrates, fats, proteins, vitamins, and minerals. (These are explained in the chapter WEIGHT CONTROL.)

On the following pages are menus for six full days which offer these basic ingredients.

Each day's selection of three meals offers a truly balanced and complete diet — in terms of nourishment, strength-building, and energy replenishment, as well as for building "stored energy" into the body while at the same time keeping it hard and trim.

# TYPICAL TRAINING TABLE MENUS

## Monday:

### Breakfast

Chilled orange-grapefruit
   juice
Chilled purple plums
Dry cereal
Eggs any style
Crisp hot toast
Butter
Honey dip doughnuts
Strawberry preserves
Coffee — milk

### Lunch

Chilled orange juice
Grilled hamburger steak
Chopped raw onions
Sliced kosher pickles
Potato chips
Sliced tomatoes — Lettuce
Mayonnaise — Dressing
Chilled pineapple rings
Cookies
Hamburger rolls — Butter
Iced tea — Coffee

### Dinner

Chilled pineapple juice
Grilled sirloin strip steak
   au jus
Whole baked Idaho potato
Fresh frozen garden peas
Head lettuce salad
Russian dressing
Raspberry gelatin
Honey
Crisp hot toast
Butter
Iced tea — Coffee — Milk

## Tuesday:

### Breakfast

Chilled pineapple sections
Chilled prune juice
Dry cereal
Eggs any style
Grilled link sausage
Hot griddle cakes
Crisp hot toast
Butter
Pancake syrup
Grape jelly
Coffee — Milk

### Lunch

Chilled tomato juice
Saltines
Baked Vienna meat loaf
Creamy whipped potatoes
Carrots and peas
Apple-celery raisin salad
Crisp bed of lettuce
Home-made cherry cobbler
Vanilla sauce
Hot pan rolls — Butter
Iced tea — Coffee

### Dinner

Old-fashioned bean soup
Saltines
Grilled center cut pork
   chops
Country-style brown gravy
Applesauce
Creamy whipped potatoes
Whole small Harvard beets
Chef's tossed garden salad
Assorted dressings
Chocolate pudding
Parker House rolls — Butter
Iced tea — Coffee — Milk

| Wednesday: | Thursday: |
|---|---|

### Wednesday:

#### *Breakfast*

Chilled tomato juice
Chilled honey dew melon
Dry cereal
Eggs any style
Rashers of bacon
Crisp hot toast
Butter
Pineapple — Apricot
   preserves
Coffee — Milk

#### *Lunch*

Chilled pineapple juice
Boston-style baked beans
Steamed frankfurters
Chopped raw onions
Sweet pickle relish
Potato chips
Chopped lettuce — Tomato
   wedges
Mayonnaise — Dressing
Strawberry gelatin —
Cream whip topping
   Cookies
Hot dog rolls — Butter
Iced tea — Coffee

#### *Dinner*

Chicken noodle soup
Saltines
Roast prime rib of beef
   au jus
Baked Idaho potato stuffed
   with Cheddar cheese
Fresh Brussels sprouts
Chef's sweet-sour salad
Sweet-sour vinegar dressing
Ice-cold watermelon
Cloverleaf rolls
Butter
Icer tea — Coffee — Milk

### Thursday:

#### *Breakfast*

Chilled grapefruit juice
Chilled Kadota figs
Dry cereal
Eggs any style
Canadian bacon
Crisp hot toast
Butter
Black cherry preserves
Coffee — Milk

#### *Lunch*

Chilled apricot nectar
Assorted cold cuts
Sweet mixed pickles
Mixed vegetables
Potato chips
German-style potato salad
Sliced tomatoes — Lettuce
Mayonnaise — Dressing
Vanilla pudding
Bread — Butter
Iced tea — Coffee

#### *Dinner*

Home-style vegetable soup
Saltines
Sirloin Swiss steak club style
Fresh vegetable gravy
Browned new potatoes
Fresh buttered succotash
Chilled pineapple rings
Cottage cheese salad
Cherry gelatin
Cookies
Whole maraschino cherry
Muffin-tin rolls — Butter
Iced tea — Coffee — Milk

## Friday:

### Breakfast

Chilled orange juice
Chilled cantaloupe
Wheaties
Eggs any style
Grilled Virginia ham
Crisp hot toast
Butter
Home-made sticky buns
Blackberry preserves
Coffee — Milk

### Lunch

Chilled pineapple juice
White meat albacore tuna
   salad
Cold sliced beef — Ham —
   Cheese
Sweet pickle chips
Diced mustard pickle
Potato sticks
Home-style macaroni salad
Sliced tomatoes — Lettuce
Mayonnaise — Dressing
Butterscotch pudding —
Cream whip topping
   Cookies
Bread — Butter
Iced tea — Coffee

### Dinner

Maryland style crab soup
Saltines
Fried filet of fresh flounder
Grilled lamb chops
Tartar sauce — Mint jelly
French-fried potatoes
Fresh buttered asparagus
Cole slaw salad
Boiled spiced dressing
Home-made peach pie
   a la mode
Parker House rolls
Butter
Iced tea — Coffee — Milk

## Saturday:

### Breakfast

Chilled pineapple juice
Diced fresh oranges
Wheaties
Eggs any style
Rashers of bacon
Crisp hot toast
Butter
Honey dip doughnuts
Peach preserves
Coffee — Milk

### Lunch

Chilled orange juice
Grilled hamburger steak
Chopped raw onions
Sliced dill chips
Potato chips
Sliced tomatoes — Lettuce
Mayonnaise — Dressing
Chocolate pudding
Cookies
Hamburger rolls — butter
Iced tea — Coffee

### Dinner

Chilled grapefruit juice
Grilled sirloin strip steak
   au jus
Whole baked Idaho potato
Fresh-frozen garden peas
Head lettuce salad
Bleu cheese dressing
Strawberry gelatin
Honey
Crisp hot toast
Butter
Iced tea — Coffee — Milk

# 13

## SLEEP, REST, AND RELAXATION

No physical fitness program can be effective without enough sleep, rest, and relaxation.

Sleep is the basic source of man's recuperative power. While you are sleeping, your body recovers from the normal wear and tear of living by repairing and replenishing your muscles, tissues, and body organs. Sleep is also "nature's way" of draining away both mental and physical tension.

The average person needs about eight hours of sleep a night, but this is highly individual. The right amount of sleep is whatever you need to wake up every morning feeling fresh, energetic, and alert. Failure to get enough sleep will lead to exhaustion, slower reflexes, and loss of endurance.

On the other extreme, there are people who consistently get *too much* sleep. As a result, they wake up with a "drugged" feeling, which they often confuse with not having slept soundly. It is a well-known fact that emotionally disturbed people often use sleep as an "escape." If you find you need more than ten hours of sleep every night, you should see a doctor.

## Rest

Rest, in a sense, is a "little sleep." Even when you do not go to sleep, you benefit from letting your body relax completely. Lying down for just 15 minutes can be a great help in clearing both your body and mind of tension and fatigue.

## Relaxation

While sleep and rest are vital to your physical well-being, relaxation is vital to your mental well-being. The essence of relaxation is *change.* Man must have variety in his life in order to maintain his zest, alertness, and optimistic outlook.

Relaxation is a broad subject, but it clearly relates to how you spend your working hours. An athlete would find relaxation in going to the movies, playing cards, or following a quiet hobby like building model ships. For this is a great *change* from his daily routine. The desk-weary businessman, on the other hand, would find relaxation in physical activity — playing golf, going swimming, or even taking a long walk.

### VACATIONS

A vacation combines the benefits of rest and relaxation.

Not only do you rest physically, but by being "away from it all" you automatically follow the path of pleasure and engage in activities which you enjoy.

A vacation — whether in the mountains, at the seashore, or in another town — is both physically restful and psychologically invigorating. It not only rests the body with a complete change of pace, but rests the mind with a complete change of scene.

## Avoid Paying the Price of Fatigue

A lack of sleep, rest, and relaxation will result in fatigue. Without enough sleep, you will suffer *body fatigue* which will cripple your vitality. This defeats the energy-building benefits of your exercise program. A lack of rest and relaxation leads to *mental fatigue,* which results in depression, listlessness, and a lack of interest in life.

Again, we emphasize that physical fitness is a "whole." It is only by blending a carefully selected program of exercises with good posture, a balanced diet, sleep, rest, and relaxation — all governed by self-discipline and common sense — that you can reach an ideal state of physical fitness in which you can enjoy life to its fullest.